2nd edition

101
Tips
for
Improving
your Blood
Sugar

University of New Mexico Diabetes Care Team

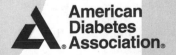

**American
Diabetes
Association.**

Book Acquisitions	Robert J. Anthony
Editor	Sherrye Landrum
Production Director	Carolyn R. Segree
Production Coordinator	Peggy M. Rote
Composition	Sherrye Landrum
Cover Design	Wickham & Associates, Inc.
Printer	Transcontinental Printing, Inc.

Printed in Canada
1 3 5 7 9 10 8 6 4 2

The suggestions and information contained in this publication are generally consistent with the Clinical Practice Recommendations and other policies of the American Diabetes Association, but they do not represent the policy or position of the Association or any of its boards or committees. Reasonable steps have been taken to ensure the accuracy of the information presented. However, the American Diabetes Association cannot ensure the safety or efficacy of any product or service described in this publication. Individuals are advised to consult a physician or other appropriate health care professional before undertaking any diet or exercise program or taking any medication referred to in this publication. Professionals must use and apply their own professional judgment, experience, and training and should not rely solely on the information contained in this publication before prescribing any diet, exercise, or medication. The American Diabetes Association—its officers, directors, employees, volunteers, and members—assumes no responsibility or liability for personal or other injury, loss, or damage that may result from the suggestions or information in this publication.

ADA titles may be purchased for business or promotional use or for special sales. For information, please write to Lee M. Romano, Special Sales & Promotions, at the address below.

American Diabetes Association
1660 Duke Street
Alexandria, Virginia 22314

Library of Congress Cataloging-in-Publication Data
101 tips for improving your blood sugar : a project of the American Diabetes Association / written and produced by The University of New Mexico Diabetes Care Team; David S. Schade, editor in chief... [et al.]. --2nd ed.
    p.   cm.
    ISBN 1–58040–026–4 pbk.
    1. Diabetes Popular works. 2. Diabetes Miscellanea. I. Schade, David S., 1942– .
II. University of New Mexico. Diabetes Care Group. III. American Diabetes Association.
IV. Title: One hundred and one tips for improving your blood sugar.   V. Title: One hundred and one tips for improving your blood sugar.

    RC660.4.A15   1999
    616.4'62—dc21   99–22929
                                                     CIP

101 TIPS FOR IMPROVING YOUR BLOOD SUGAR

▼

TABLE OF CONTENTS

Acknowledgments

▼

The University of New Mexico Diabetes Care Team wishes to acknowledge the talent, graphic design, and desktop publishing skills of Paul Akmajian, MFA, of the University of New Mexico. His skills brought this book to life. We also acknowledge the editorial assistance of Sherrye Landrum of the American Diabetes Association, the assistance of Carolyn King, MEd, of the University of New Mexico, and the graphic expertise of Steve Rhodes of Insight Graphics. Thanks to Karen Ingle for copyediting both editions of this book and to David Kelley, MD; Linda Lacey, RN, CDE; and Patti B. Geil, MS, RD, FADA, CDE, for reviewing the manuscript. Steve Shartel coordinated the first printing, and Peggy Rote handled the printing of the second edition.

Introduction

▼

The treatment of diabetes has dramatically changed in the past five years. No longer is it acceptable to permit blood sugar to remain above normal in a person with diabetes. The medical consequences of high blood sugar are largely preventable when blood sugar is kept in normal ranges.

During the last 10 years, we have been fortunate to care for many people with diabetes who made the commitment to improve their blood sugar levels. Most of these individuals have achieved their goals and, in addition, told us how they did it. This book is a collection of their suggestions and experiences that we are passing on to you. We hope that many of these tips will apply to your lifestyle and help you control your blood sugar more easily.

We have revised this book to be certain that all tips are current. Diabetes care changes rapidly, and new information becomes available daily. We have replaced out-of-date tips, added graphics, and given you an extra 10 tips to provide you with the newest information.

—The University of New Mexico Diabetes Care Team

Chapter 1
GENERAL TIPS

How do I know whether I have type 1 or type 2 diabetes?

▼
TIP:

With type 1 diabetes the body stops making insulin. This usually occurs at a young age. People with type 1 diabetes will require insulin for life because insulin is essential for using and storing food. These people are usually lean and, if they did not have insulin, would go into diabetic coma within a day or two. In the past, this disease was called insulin-dependent diabetes mellitus (IDDM). The proper name is now type 1 diabetes.

People with type 2 diabetes have enough insulin early in the disease, but their bodies are unable to use the insulin correctly to lower blood sugar. They are *insulin resistant*. Many people with type 2 diabetes are able to control their blood sugar with diet and exercise, and some take oral diabetes pills. In the past, this type of diabetes was called non-insulin-dependent diabetes mellitus (NIDDM). The correct term is now type 2 diabetes. After several years with type 2 diabetes, many people will need insulin, but they still have type 2 diabetes, insulin-requiring. Most people with type 2 diabetes are overweight and more than 30 years old.

If I didn't have diabetes, what would my normal blood sugar be?

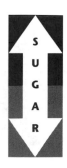

TIP:

The answer to this question depends on whether you have eaten food in the last 6 hours. Before breakfast, when you have not had food for 8 or more hours, normal blood sugar would be between 70 and 105 mg/dl. However, after a meal, normal blood sugar rarely goes above 200 mg/dl. People who do not have diabetes don't have problems associated with high blood sugar (diabetic complications). That is why your blood sugar goal is to stay close to the upper limit of normal blood sugar ranges.

NORMAL BLOOD GLUCOSE LEVELS

Fasting blood glucose	<105 mg/dl
After meal blood glucose (2-h)	140 mq/dl
Bedtime glucose	<120 mg/dl
Hemoglobin A$_{1c}$	<6%

< means less than

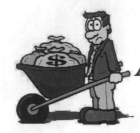

As a resident of the United States, how much does diabetes cost me?

▼
TIP:

In the United States, total medical costs to care for diabetes in 1997 were approximately $98 billion. These costs are usually divided into two parts, direct medical costs and indirect costs. Direct medical costs are those that are paid directly for either hospitalization, nursing, or treatment at home. Indirect costs are costs from a diabetes-caused disability such that a person cannot go back to work or from premature death and loss of a productive citizen. On a per person basis, health care for a person with diabetes costs approximately $10,000 per patient per year compared with $2,600 for people who do not have diabetes. In other words, health care for a person with diabetes costs four times as much as health care for a person without diabetes. This is one reason why great emphasis is placed on preventing diabetes and improving the treatment of patients to prevent diabetic complications.

*W̶hat are my blood sugar goals if I have
diabetes?*

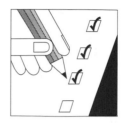

▼
TIP:

W̶e encourage you to try for nearly normal blood sugar levels
with few episodes of low blood sugar. The American Diabetes Association (ADA) goals are listed below. If you are persis-
tently outside of these goals or have low blood sugar too often, you
need to discuss changing your diabetes therapy with your health
care team. These goals are determined from studies that examined
the effects of near-normal blood sugar levels on the rates of diabetic
complications.

BLOOD SUGAR GOALS FOR PEOPLE WITH DIABETES (mg/dl)

	Normal	Good	Action Needed
Before meal blood sugar	<110	80–120	<80 or >200
After meal	<120	200	<100 or >160
Hemoglobin A$_{1c}$	<6%	7%	8%

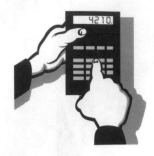

*H*ow can I tell if my diabetes program is successful?

▼
TIP:

K eep track of your diabetes the same way you do your checking account—by keeping tabs on the balance. With diabetes, the balance is the sum of
- Your blood sugar
- Your daily weight
- Your blood pressure
- Your exercise
- How you feel

If all of these items meet your goals, then you are doing fine.

Keep a daily record of your blood glucose and weight. You can check your blood pressure at home or have it done at shopping centers, pharmacies, etc. Make daily exercise one of your goals. When you monitor your health daily, you help yourself succeed.

EXAMPLE RECORD

Date	Wt	Blood Pressure	Average Glucose	Feelings	Exercise
6/1	150	122/80	102	Good	Yes
6/2	151	120/75	111	Good	No
6/3	149	115/80	98	So/So	Yes

What determines when type 1 diabetes develops?

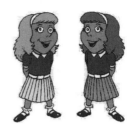

▼
TIP:

We don't understand all of the factors that lead to type 1 diabetes. Until very recently, it was believed that type 1 diabetes did not occur in susceptible individuals until they were exposed to some specific environmental trigger that initiated an immune response against the insulin-producing cells of the pancreas. Years later, when almost all of the insulin-producing cells were destroyed, diabetes would develop. Possible trigger events include viral infections or drinking cow's milk as an infant. A recent study, however, suggests that genetics may have more to do with when type 1 diabetes develops than was previously thought. Scientists compared the age at onset of type 1 diabetes among a group of identical twins to groups of nonidentical twins and non-twin siblings who also had diabetes. The study showed that the development of type 1 diabetes in one identical twin predicted the development of type 1 diabetes in the other twin much more accurately than when one nonidentical twin or non-twin sibling developed type 1 diabetes. Because identical twins are genetically identical, this study suggests that genetics plays a stronger role than previously thought in the development of type 1 diabetes.

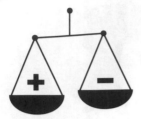

If I follow all the advice in this book and my blood sugar control improves, are there drawbacks that I should be aware of?

▼
TIP:

Yes, there are. However, these are usually not bad enough to discourage you from keeping your blood sugar near normal. The two main concerns are frequent episodes of low blood sugar and a tendency to gain weight. You can head off low blood sugar by monitoring carefully. You can keep your weight in line by watching the number of calories you eat and by increasing the amount of exercise you do. Overall, the disadvantages are minor compared to the benefits you gain from lowering your blood sugar.

Why should I work so hard to improve my blood sugar level?

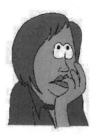

▼
TIP:

Because you'll feel more energy and a greater sense of well-being when your blood sugar enters the normal range. In addition, you'll delay or prevent problems with your eyes, kidneys, and nerves as your blood sugar improves. Many doctors also believe that problems with heart discase, strokes, and hardening of the arteries may be delayed by good blood sugar control. If you do not get any complications of diabetes, you'll live a longer, healthier life.

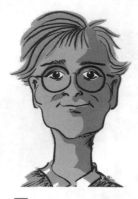

Will controlling my blood sugar prevent my recently diagnosed diabetic eye disease from getting worse?

▼
TIP:

Yes. Although improving your blood sugar control may temporarily make your eye disease worse, over the long term, it will help. The Diabetes Control and Complications Trial (DCCT) monitored patients with mild diabetic eye disease for years. This study showed that the diabetic eye disease of patients with good blood sugar control progressed much more slowly than the eye disease of similar patients with poor blood sugar control. This is a major reason to strive for excellent blood sugar control, particularly if you have mild to moderate complications of diabetes. Another long-term study called the United Kingdom Prospective Diabetes Study (UKPDS) focused on people with type 2 diabetes and found the same beneficial effects of good blood sugar control.

*D*o I have to use alcohol on my finger before checking my blood sugar like the nurses at the hospital do?

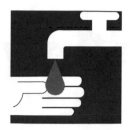

TIP:

No. Using alcohol is not necessary before checking your sugar level. Washing and drying your hands is enough. Just be sure that there is no soap left on your hands and they are dry. Test strips for determining the glucose (blood sugar) in your blood have a substance in them that causes sugar to turn into a colored chemical. Alcohol can destroy this substance and cause a false low blood sugar reading. Alcohol is drying and can lead to broken skin near nails. Also, if all the alcohol doesn't evaporate before you stick your finger, you may feel stinging as well as the discomfort of the poke.

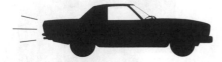

How should I prepare for a long car trip alone so I don't get high or low blood sugars?

▼
TIP:

The best way to approach a long driving trip alone is to establish a routine. Start your day early so that you can arrive at your destination early. Because you are less active while driving, exercise before you leave or stop along the way at a park or rest area and take a walk. You might also consider either slightly increasing your daily insulin or decreasing the amount of food that you eat. Because hypoglycemia (low blood sugar) is particularly dangerous when you are driving, plan on checking your blood sugar levels frequently (every 2 to 4 hours) and always have some form of sugar in the car with you. Choose something that won't melt and be messy, such as glucose tablets, a bottle of regular soda, or vanilla wafers.

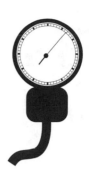

Why did my doctor recently start me on a blood pressure medication even though my blood pressure is only slightly elevated?

▼
TIP:

High blood sugar combined with high blood pressure increases your risk of getting diabetic kidney disease. Kidney disease can lead to kidney failure and the need for either dialysis or a kidney transplant. Doctors can identify diabetic kidney disease at a very early stage, when small amounts of protein appear in the urine (microalbuminuria). Certain drugs that lower blood pressure, such as ACE inhibitors, also lower microalbuminuria and can slow down the development of kidney disease. A lower protein diet may also be beneficial in preventing kidney problems.

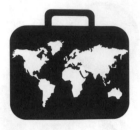

*W*hat if my blood glucose meter quits
working while I am on an out-of-town
trip?

TIP:

Continue monitoring your blood sugar with visual test strips (Chemstrip, Diascan, Glucostix). These are available without a prescription at most pharmacies. In the meantime, call the toll-free number that can usually be found on the back of the meter. Most companies will try to replace the meter within a day or two.

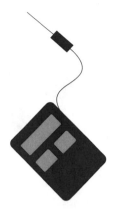

*W*ill an insulin pump improve my
blood sugar control?

TIP:

Maybe, maybe not. It depends on the individual. These devices require you to pay close attention to your blood sugar levels and to adjust your insulin, food, and exercise to achieve good readings. With an insulin pump, you can vary your mealtime schedule more readily than with insulin injections, and you can skip a meal when you must. There is more flexibility for people with unpredictable mealtimes. Discuss the pros and cons of using an insulin pump and whether you are a good candidate for having one with your health care team before purchasing one. Also, because they are expensive, check whether your insurance company will help cover the cost.

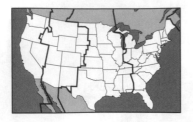

*H*ow do I make adjustments in my insulin when I travel across several time zones?

▼
TIP:

The easiest approach is to omit your intermediate- or long-acting insulin on the morning of the trip and rely on regular insulin to keep your blood sugar normal. You will have to test your blood sugar frequently (every 4 hours) and take regular insulin frequently (every 4 hours, adjusting the insulin dose to your blood sugar level). When you arrive at your destination and change your watch to the new time zone, go back on your usual insulin and meal schedule.

*I*s there a level of average blood sugar below which I do not have to worry about complications from diabetes?

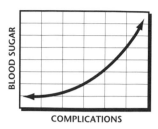

▼
TIP:

No. There is no safe threshold. The DCCT looked at the relationship between average blood sugar levels (as measured by hemoglobin A_{1c}) and the beginning of complications. There is no level below which the risk disappears. However, the lower your hemoglobin A_{1c}, the lower your risk of eye, kidney, and nerve disease. Therefore, you should try for the best average blood sugar that you can (but still avoid seriously low blood sugars) to reduce your risk of having diabetic complications.

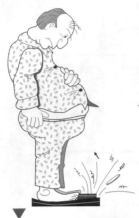

*H*ow does the fact that I am overweight affect
my ability to obtain normal blood sugars?

▼
TIP:

Being overweight causes resistance to insulin. This means that
any insulin that your body may make (or that you inject) will
have a hard time lowering your blood sugar. This makes it difficult
for you to control your blood sugar. In addition, being overweight
may raise your blood pressure, which makes you prone to kidney
disease and stroke. Being overweight may also be associated with
high blood fat levels, which makes you susceptible to hardening of
the arteries. If you reduce your weight, your blood sugar levels and
your health will improve.

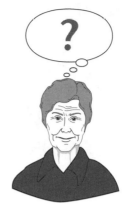

*A*t age 72, why should I worry about blood sugar control?

▼
TIP:

Age alone is not a reason to ignore your diabetes control. You may live to be 90 or 100 years old. This is enough time for complications of diabetes to develop. The better your blood sugar control, the lower your risk of developing complications.

   People are lowering their risk of diabetic complications through intensive diabetes management. They do have more frequent low blood sugars, but that is riskier for some people than for others. People with heart disease and people who do not feel warning signs when they develop low blood sugar (for example, shakiness, sweating, or increased heart rate) need to be careful. People who live alone also need to be careful. Tight blood sugar control is not for everyone (and may even be dangerous for some). You and your health care team should determine what blood sugar levels are right for you.

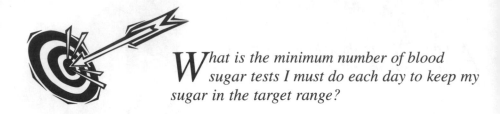

What is the minimum number of blood sugar tests I must do each day to keep my sugar in the target range?

▼
TIP:

The answer depends on the type of diabetes you have. Most people with type 1 diabetes and people with type 2 who require insulin need to test their blood sugar four times a day (before each meal and at bedtime) to allow them to adjust their premeal insulin dose. People with type 2 diabetes may need to test only before breakfast each day. Occasionally, people with type 1 or type 2 diabetes should test their blood sugar 2 to 3 hours after a meal to find out whether it is going too high or in the middle of the night to see whether it is going too low. If so, the amount of food, exercise, or medication may need to be adjusted. All people with diabetes should test their blood sugar any time they think it may be too high or too low. The symptoms of being high or low may be similar (see p. 25), or these symptoms may not be due to blood sugar at all!

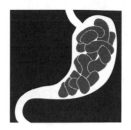

*W*ill my blood glucose be affected if my stomach empties slowly?

▼
TIP:

Yes. If it takes many hours for your stomach to empty and food to be absorbed after a meal, you risk low blood sugar when you take your insulin 45 minutes before you eat. The insulin will peak before the food is absorbed, and you may have high blood sugar many hours later when your stomach finally empties. The common cause of slowed digestion in people who have had diabetes for many years is damage to the nerves affecting stomach muscle activity. This condition is called gastroparesis. Unpredictable stomach emptying makes it difficult to achieve near-normal blood sugars. There are several medications now available that may improve the motion of your stomach, and you should discuss these with your health care team.

Chapter 2
HIGH BLOOD SUGAR
TIPS

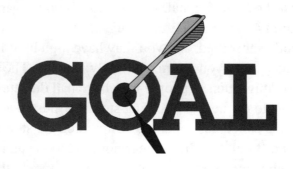

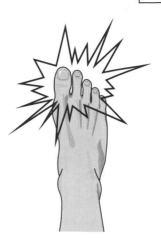

*D*oes the pain in my feet have anything to do with high blood sugar?

▼
TIP:

Probably, especially if you have had high blood sugar for many years, and the pain has lasted for several months. Nerves work better when they are surrounded by normal rather than high blood sugar. Discuss your pain with your health care team. Some people find the pain in their feet and legs will decrease when their blood sugar is brought closer to normal. Others find it painful for bed-sheets to touch their feet. If you experience this, placing a hoop over the end of the bed so that the sheet is kept off of your feet will provide relief until your blood sugars can be lowered. If the problem doesn't go away with improved blood sugar control, then putting capsaicin cream (which is made from chili peppers) on the affected skin may help. Other therapies (especially medication) are also available, so you need to discuss the various choices with your diabetes health care team.

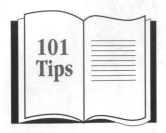

I have read this book, so why do I need help from anyone else to control my high blood sugars?

▼
TIP:

Although books on diabetes have many good, helpful suggestions to control your blood sugar, there are many situations in which you need additional advice. Your doctor and health care team can

1. Help you choose the blood sugar goal that is appropriate for you
2. Teach you how to care for your diabetes and keep you up to date on new treatments
3. Help you develop a meal plan
4. Check your medications so they don't interfere with each other
5. Design a physical activity program specifically for you
6. Review your blood sugar records with you and make suggestions on how to improve your sugar control
7. Help you manage your diabetes when you become ill and thereby prevent more serious health problems

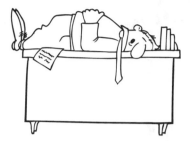

*W*hat are the symptoms of
high blood sugar?

▼
TIP:

Symptoms of high blood sugar may vary from person to person
or even in one person from day to day. But, in general, a person
will
1. Feel more hungry or thirsty than usual
2. Have to urinate more frequently than normal
3. Have to get up at night several times to go to the bathroom
4. Feel very tired or sleepy or have no energy
5. Be unable to see clearly or see "halos" when looking at a light
   If you have any of the above symptoms, locate your glucose
meter and check immediately. Do not treat these symptoms with
additional insulin unless you are certain that they are due to high
blood sugar. There are other conditions that cause similar symptoms.

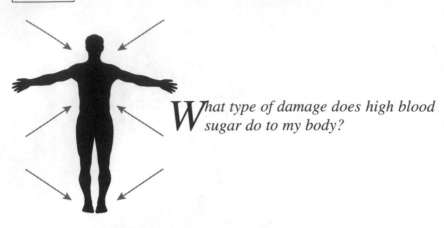

What type of damage does high blood sugar do to my body?

▼
TIP:

Over time, high blood sugar levels can damage both blood vessels and nerves in your body. This can result in poor blood flow to your hands and feet in addition to your legs, arms, and vital organs. Poor blood flow to these areas increases your risk of infections, heart problems, stroke, blindness, foot or leg amputation, and kidney disease. In addition, you can either lose the feeling in your feet or have increased pain in your feet and legs. Damage to your feet can occur from mild injuries, and you may not know it. Finally, damage to blood vessels and nerves can lead to sexual problems that are difficult to treat. For all these reasons, you should make a major effort to avoid high blood sugars in your body.

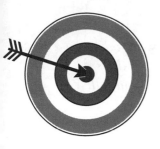

Why is my glycosylated hemoglobin high when my average blood sugar is in my target range?

▼
TIP:

Your average blood sugar is probably based on your premeal blood sugars. While this usually works well, it does not take into account the level of your blood sugar after you eat. It may be that your blood sugar is rising unexpectedly after your meal because you are either not taking enough insulin or not taking insulin far enough ahead of eating your meal. To see if this is the reason that your glycosylated hemoglobin is high, measure your blood sugar 2 hours after breakfast, lunch, and dinner for several days (in addition to your premeal blood sugars). Blood sugar that is more than 200 mg/dl 2 hours after a meal is too high. In addition, your blood sugar may be high throughout the night, when you are asleep. To find out, wake yourself up at 4:00 A.M. several times during the week to check your blood sugar. At 4:00 A.M., blood sugar that is higher than 150 mg/dl is too high. Continue to check your blood sugar 2 hours after meals and in the middle of the night once a month to be certain that you are not having unexpected high blood sugars at these times.

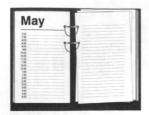

How can I evaluate my blood sugar control when my doctor does a hemoglobin A₁c only every 6 months?

▼
TIP:

You can use your self-monitored blood glucose results to predict your hemoglobin A_{1c} (HbA$_{1c}$). Here's how. Average all your blood sugar check results each week. Find your average on the table below. Read across to the HbA$_{1c}$ number. This will give you an idea of your HbA$_{1c}$ range, before your doctor measures it. Your blood sugar ranges might be slightly different if the normal range of your laboratory's HbA$_{1c}$ is different from ours. Our normal range of HbA$_{1c}$ is 4.5–6.5%. Find out your laboratory's normal HbA$_{1c}$ range and use it to revise this table. If you have type 1 diabetes, have an HbA$_{1c}$ test done every 3 months.

Average Glucose (mg/dl)	Predicted HbA$_{1c}$
<100	<6.5
100–120	6.5–7.0
120–140	7.0–7.5
140–160	7.5–8.0
160–180	8.0–8.5
>180	>8.5

*W*hy would my blood sugar be high
before supper when I use regular
insulin before each meal and NPH at
night?

▼
TIP:

Average doses of regular insulin last only 4 to 6 hours. Because the time between lunch and supper can often be 6 or 7 hours, it is not surprising that your lunchtime insulin is wearing off before supper.

An ideal insulin regimen is flexible to allow for whatever changes come up in your day-to-day schedule. You should be able to make adjustments to correct for unusual swings in your blood sugar that result from known or unknown causes. The regimen you describe is very popular, but many people find that not having an intermediate- or long-acting insulin during the day limits how flexible they can be. As you can see, your regimen is not dealing with the blood sugar rise before supper. Talk to your health care team about this pattern you see developing, so they can suggest ways to prevent it.

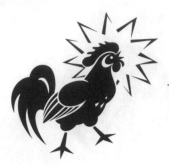

Why are my morning blood sugars usually the highest of the day?

▼
TIP:

The reason for high morning blood sugars may be related to how long your insulin covers your body's needs overnight. In many people, human NPH is too short-acting because it may last only 6–8 hours. This may not be long enough to maintain good blood sugar levels overnight if you take your NPH at suppertime. Try moving your evening NPH injection to bedtime. If this change doesn't work, however, then you need to consider switching to a longer-acting insulin, such as human ultralente. Many people who use two injections of human ultralente per day (in addition to regular insulin before each meal) see improvement in their morning blood sugars. Or you may need to increase your dose. To see if you have nighttime lows, check your blood sugar between 2:00 and 4:00 A.M. Starting off the day with a blood sugar close to normal is a key to good overall blood sugar control.

APPROXIMATE INSULIN ACTION

	Onset	Peak	Duration
Lispro	<15 min	0.5–1.5 h	2–4 h
Regular	0.5–1 h	2–3 h	4–10 h
NPH	2–4 h	5–9 h	10–16 h
Lente	3–4 h	4–12 h	12–18 h
Ultralente	6–10 h	—	18–24 h

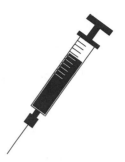

Should I take large doses of regular insulin when my blood sugar is high?

▼
TIP:

For an adult, very high blood sugars do not necessarily require very large doses of regular or lispro insulin. While it makes sense to increase your insulin when your blood sugar is high, increasing your regular dose by 1 or 2 units is unlikely to make your blood sugar come down much faster. In fact, the main effect of taking larger dosages of regular insulin is that the insulin works over a longer period of time. For example, a large morning dose of regular insulin may result in mid-afternoon hypoglycemia. If you are using lispro insulin, you may be able to bring your sugar down faster by taking a larger dose, but you may also have mid-afternoon hypoglycemia. Thus, if you are using regular insulin, when your blood sugars are very high,

1. Take your regular insulin dose immediately.

2. Drink large amounts of water to stay well hydrated.

3. Delay your next meal until your blood sugar is below 200 mg/dl. This may mean waiting 1 or 2 hours (or more) after injecting your insulin before eating.

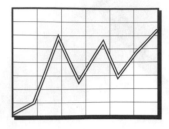

Why do my blood sugar levels vary so much since I switched to ultralente insulin?

TIP:

One of the reasons may be because you do not always get the same concentration of insulin crystals into the syringe. One basic instruction that is often overlooked when patients start on ultralente insulin is how to mix the crystals correctly. After you rock the bottle between your palms, you must immediately draw the dose out of the bottle. The weight and shape of these crystals cause them to settle rapidly back to the bottom of the bottle. If you set the bottle down to draw your regular insulin and then return to the ultralente, the amount of insulin suspended may be quite different from that in the dose you drew up immediately.

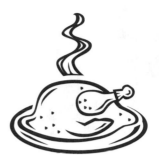

*W hat should I do when it's getting
close to my meal time and my
blood sugar is above 240 mg/dl?*

▼
TIP:

High blood sugar before a meal tells you that your liver is making too much glucose and needs to be told to slow down! The
signal it needs is insulin. Because it takes time for insulin to be
absorbed from the skin and additional time to reduce the liver's glucose production, we suggest that you take your usual dose of insulin
and wait 60–90 minutes (instead of the usual 30–45 minutes) to eat.
This will allow your blood sugar level to fall toward the normal
range before you eat, giving the insulin a "head start." The goal is
not to become low before eating but to regain control over high
blood sugar. An alternative is to take lispro insulin 15–30 minutes
before your meal, which should lower your blood sugar more rapidly than regular insulin.

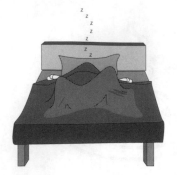

*H*ow *can I sleep late on weekends without waking up with high blood sugar?*

▼
TIP:

If you want to sleep late (for example, until 10:00 or 11:00 in the morning), then set your alarm for 6:00 A.M., go to the bathroom, and check your blood sugar. If your blood sugar is high, take 2–4 units of regular insulin so that while you are sleeping late, your blood sugar will slowly decline. If your blood sugar is low, you should drink some juice or milk. If your blood sugar is normal, take 1 or 2 units of regular insulin and go back to sleep. This schedule has worked well for many people, and often they do not even remember waking up at 6:00 A.M. and taking their insulin.

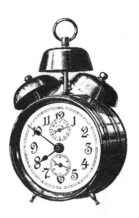

*H*ow soon after I wake up in the morning should I check my blood sugar?

▼
TIP:

Check your blood sugar immediately on awakening—before any morning activities, such as showering, shaving, or putting on makeup. The reason for this schedule is that if your blood sugar is low, you can drink some juice or milk. If it is high, you can take your insulin immediately and allow it to work at least 1 hour before breakfast. It is important to get into this habit, because if you start the day with a normal blood sugar level before breakfast, keeping your blood sugar under control throughout the day is much easier. Monitoring your sugar immediately on awakening does not take a major change in lifestyle, but it is very effective in improving your blood sugar control.

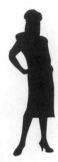

Why do my blood sugars run high before I have my menstrual period?

▼
TIP:

Many women with diabetes have swings in blood sugar control around the time of menstruation. There are many possible reasons for this, from changes in behavior (eating more food) to hormonal changes (high estrogen levels before the period begins can increase your insulin requirements). Young women seem to have the largest swings in blood sugar during their monthly cycle and need to adjust their insulin. Older women also have erratic swings in hormone levels and may have a challenge with maintaining blood sugar control. As you become familiar with your body's rhythm, you may find that the changes in your insulin needs become predictable from month to month. Monitor your blood sugar often and adjust your insulin as necessary during your menstrual period.

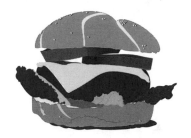

Why do I get high sugars after I treat a low blood sugar reaction?

▼
TIP:

Two factors raise your blood sugar after a low blood sugar reaction. First, the hormones that your body naturally releases into your blood to combat low sugar slowly raise the level of blood sugar. Second, the food you eat raises your blood sugar. Many people with diabetes eat or drink too much after a low blood sugar reading. Low blood sugar causes intense hunger. All of these factors can cause high sugars 2–4 hours or longer after eating. It's important to drink only a small amount (1/2 glass) of juice or milk, or eat glucose tablets, and then recheck your blood sugar in 30 minutes. If you eat a larger amount of food, then cover the food with extra regular insulin.

Chapter 3
LOW BLOOD SUGAR TIPS

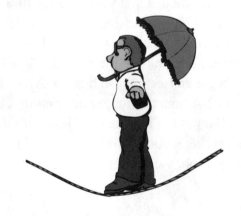

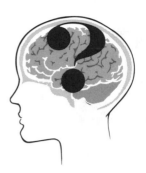

*W*ill repeated low blood sugars
  damage my ability to think
clearly?

▼
TIP:

W e don't know. A recent large study of people with repeated
     moderate low blood sugars did not show a decrease in the
brain's functioning. But low blood sugar levels can be dangerous,
particularly if they are very low or last for a prolonged period of
time. The brain uses blood sugar for energy, and if it is without fuel
for longer than a few minutes, it can suffer damage. For this reason,
treat low blood sugars rapidly, so that no damage occurs. Take special care to quickly treat low blood sugar in children to avoid damage to their growing brains.

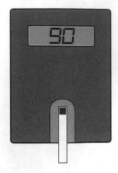

Why do I feel like my blood sugar is low when my meter says it is normal?

▼
TIP:

There are several possibilities. First, your glucose meter may be broken, dirty, or the battery may be low. Repair it, clean it, and change the battery. (Call the manufacturer if you need help.) Have your health care team check the accuracy of your meter.

Second, it takes several weeks for you to get used to normal blood sugars when you have had high blood sugars for a long period of time. Your body may be sending you false signals.

Third, you can feel like your blood sugar is low if your blood sugar rapidly drops from a high level to a normal level. This usually occurs after a large dose of regular insulin. For all these reasons, don't guess what your blood sugar is—always measure it.

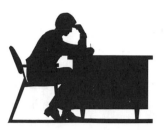

*W*hy did I have a low blood sugar this morning even though I didn't eat anything different and took my usual insulin dose?

TIP:

Exercise can sometimes result in low blood sugar that night or the next day. This is called "delayed onset low blood sugar." A day of skiing or 18 holes of golf can result in low blood sugar during your sleep that night or even the next day. Whenever you exercise strenuously, it's a good idea to check your blood sugar more frequently. Eat extra carbohydrates as needed during the next 24 hours or adjust your insulin dose.

Another factor is that intermediate- or long-acting insulin is absorbed at different rates from day to day. For example, injecting into your leg and then exercising can cause the insulin to be absorbed more quickly than usual. You can control this to some extent by injecting insulin into the abdominal area, because it is absorbed more evenly there.

A third factor may be that you forgot your nighttime snack. This snack is important to provide early morning sugar because the food you eat for supper is usually completely absorbed by 3:00 A.M.

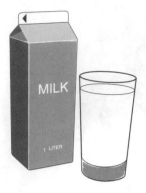

B *esides glucose tablets (which I find too sweet) and juice (which I'm tired of), what other choices do I have to treat low blood sugar reactions?*

▼
TIP:

O ne of our favorite recommended treatments is a glass of milk. Milk contains lactose that is broken down into glucose (sugar). It also has fat and protein in it to slow down the rise in your blood sugar and keep it steady over time. For this reason, milk is better than juice or glucose tablets. Fat-free and reduced-fat milk have the same amount of lactose. Other studies have found that a small amount of ice cream will work nearly as well. You might also consider graham crackers, which are easy to keep on hand. Try to avoid high-fat treatments, such as candy bars, because they aren't absorbed as quickly, may lead to very high blood sugar levels in the hours after you eat them, and can contribute to weight gain, too.

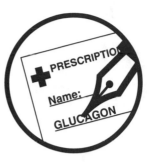

How do I protect myself against low blood sugar while I am trying for tight diabetes management?

▼
TIP:

Keep glucagon handy for emergency treatment of severe low blood sugar. If it is not an emergency, food is better and cheaper (see previous tip). Glucagon raises blood sugar. In many ways, it does the opposite of what insulin does. You get glucagon from the pharmacy with a prescription from your doctor. Someone in your household must know how to mix up the glucagon and inject it if you become severely hypoglycemic, confused, and unable to swallow food. This will need to be done quickly. Glucagon will raise your blood sugar within 10–15 minutes, but its effect doesn't last long. Eat some crackers after you become fully conscious again. Some people are nauseated after receiving glucagon. Most severe episodes of low blood sugar happen during your sleep, so to prevent your family from having to search for the glucagon, keep it in one place, such as the refrigerator door.

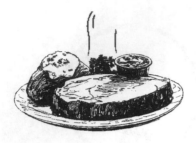

Should I take my insulin before I eat even if my blood sugar is low?

▼
TIP:

First treat the low blood sugar level with enough food to return your blood sugar to the normal range. Liquids, rather than solids, are most rapidly absorbed, and you need to drink just enough to return your blood sugar to normal. In 10–15 minutes, take your insulin and wait about 20 minutes before eating your meal. While this takes some will power, it prevents your blood sugar from rebounding and ending up above your goal of a normal blood sugar level after a meal.

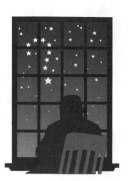

*W*hat should I do to overcome my
fear of having a low blood sugar
reaction while I'm asleep?

▼
TIP:

Many people are insecure about sleeping after having a bad time with low blood sugar during the night. It is reasonable to feel fearful. Many factors influence your blood sugar levels during the night, including how low your blood sugar level is before you go to sleep, hours worked, exercise you did during the day, changes in your insulin dose, and whether you ate or skipped a nighttime snack. If you and your physician are unable to determine why the reaction happened, try setting your alarm to wake you at 3:00 A.M. several nights in a row. If you find that your blood glucose usually falls during the night, you and your health care provider can adjust your evening insulin dose or bedtime snack. You might ask your provider about whether to try a slow-release carbohydrate snack bar, such as Zbar or Nite Bite.

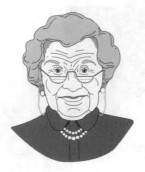

Should my 85-year-old mother try to keep her blood sugar near 150 mg/dl instead of near the normal level of 100 mg/dl?

▼
TIP:

Maybe. She and her health care team need to decide that. Each patient using intensified diabetes management has an individual blood glucose goal aimed at preventing the long-term complications of diabetes. However, asking people to come close to normal increases their risk of severe hypoglycemia (episodes of very low blood sugar). Elderly people suffer more from low blood sugars. In fact, it may increase their risk for a heart attack or cause a stroke. For some elderly people with diabetes, the risks may outweigh the benefits of trying for normal blood sugar levels. While 150 mg/dl is not a normal glucose concentration, it does offer your mother some room for her blood glucose to fall into the normal range with less fear of having serious low blood sugar.

I live alone; what can I do to reduce
the risk of a severe nighttime low
blood sugar reaction?

▼
TIP:

S tudies have shown that 50% of severe low blood sugars happen
between midnight and 8:00 A.M. (usually at 4:00 A.M.) Having a
normal blood sugar level before you go to sleep does not guarantee
that it won't drop too low a few hours later, especially if you use
intensified insulin treatments, such as nighttime NPH. Test your
blood sugar level before bed and have a good bedtime snack to prevent low blood sugar before 8:00 A.M. If nighttime low blood sugars
happen often, set your alarm and check your blood sugar level at
3:00 A.M. every night. Eat some food if it is below 75 mg/dl. Ask
your health care provider whether a slow-release carbohydrate snack
bar, such as Zbar or Nite Bite, would be a good nighttime snack for
you.

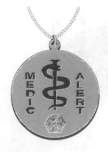

*W*hat should I do about very severe low blood sugar episodes that cause me to pass out?

▼
TIP:

Teach your family members and friends the signs and symptoms of low blood sugar, so they can help you in case you are not alert enough to tell them that your blood sugar is low. Some common symptoms are feeling shaky or lightheaded, having a rapid heartbeat, sweating, being nauseated, being confused, and having slurred speech or delayed reflexes. For those times when you may be someplace where no one knows you, carry a card in your wallet or wear a bracelet or necklace stating that you have diabetes. The card should also state whether you are on insulin and that you may become confused when you have low blood sugar. In this way, you may get help more quickly.

Work with your health care team to try to determine why you are having these episodes of low blood sugar. Keep glucagon at home or with you, and be sure a family member or friend knows how to inject it for you.

Always check your blood sugar level before you drive.

*W*hy *is my blood sugar still high*
this evening when my low blood
sugar occurred early this morning?

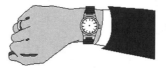

▼
TIP:

Y our body reacts to low blood sugars by secreting several hormones, including growth hormone and cortisol. These hormones may not act immediately, but after several hours, they will
raise your blood sugar. Their activity may last up to 24 hours, so you
may then have to take additional insulin to keep your blood sugar
from going too high. This rebound effect is one reason why you
want to avoid very low blood sugars. Another reason for the high
blood sugar may be that you ate too much when you tried to treat the
low blood sugar reaction.

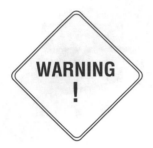

Why do I no longer feel the warning signs of low blood sugar?

TIP:

Many people who have had diabetes for more than 5 years lose some of the symptoms of low blood sugar. The usual feelings of hunger, sweatiness, anxiety, and increased heart rate may fade and escape your attention. Sometimes you may just feel sleepy as your blood sugar drops. The reasons for this are complex but are related to a loss of adrenaline release by your body when your blood sugar is low. If you are unaware of low blood sugars, try not to let your blood sugar level drop below 100 mg/dl. You may need to monitor your blood glucose levels more often.

If this is a problem for you, always check your blood sugar level before you drive.

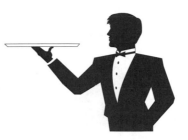

*W*hy do I develop low blood
sugar after a fancy restaurant
meal?

TIP:

Perhaps you prepare for a restaurant meal by injecting extra insulin. Restaurant meals are usually rich in fat and protein, but these nutrients do not raise your blood sugar levels as quickly as carbohydrates do, and they don't require any extra insulin. In fact, a problem with restaurant meals is getting enough carbohydrates. To increase the carbohydrate content, eat well during the bread course at the start of the meal (you might need to avoid the butter), and consider ordering a glass of skim milk with your meal or having a nonfat dessert, such as fresh fruit, or a frozen dish, such as sherbet or sorbet.

If you have an alcoholic drink when you eat out, the alcohol may be causing the low blood sugar, particularly if you eat a very small meal.

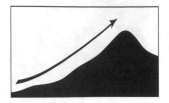

Why do my blood sugars read lower on my glucose meter when I travel from Miami (sea level) to Albuquerque (5,000 foot elevation)?

▼
TIP:

Most blood glucose meters use a chemical reaction that requires oxygen from the air to measure your blood sugar. At high altitudes, there is less oxygen in the air, which causes the results to be lower. Thus, the results you get may be affected by altitude. You should read the instructions that came with your meter and also read the package insert in the strips. You may also call the toll-free 800 number given in your package insert or write to the company that makes your meter to find out whether its readings are affected by altitude.

Chapter 4
INSULIN TIPS

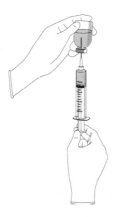

If you have type 2 diabetes, but you are taking insulin, these tips will work for you as well.

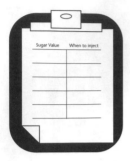

*I*s there a chart I can use to know how to time my insulin injections with my meals?

TIP:

Here is a schedule we provide to our patients with diabetes. The timing depends on your current blood sugar. In general, regular insulin should be taken 45 minutes before the meal if your sugar is high and at the meal if your sugar is low. Proper timing of the injection is also important for lispro insulin. Using this table should improve your after-meal blood sugar levels.

WHEN TO INJECT

If blood sugar value 45 minutes before meal is:	Inject Regular	Inject Lispro
<50 mg/dl	at mealtime	at end of meal
50–70 mg/dl	at mealtime	at mealtime
70–120 mg/dl	15 min before meal	at mealtime
120–180 mg/dl	30 min before meal	at mealtime
>180 mg/dl	45 min before meal	15–30 min before meal

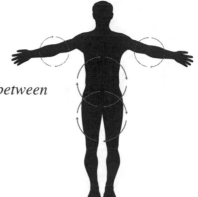

Should I rotate my insulin injection between my arms, my legs, and abdomen?

▼
TIP:

Maybe not. True, rotating your insulin injections helps you avoid always injecting into the exact same spot on your body. You don't want to do that because insulin causes local deposits of fat under the skin. However, insulin is absorbed at different speeds when it is injected into different areas of the body. Good blood sugar levels depend on you knowing how quickly your insulin will act. That is why we say to rotate your injection sites in one general area—that is, arms, or legs, or around the abdomen, but not all three. You could give your morning shots in one area and your evening shots in another area. This provides you with more predictable insulin absorption and improved blood sugar control. We suggest using the abdomen as an injection site because insulin is absorbed more rapidly in this location. Interestingly, rotation of injection sites is more important with regular insulin than with lispro insulin. In fact, site rotation has been proved to have little or no effect on the absorption of lispro insulin.

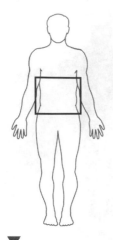

*W**here should I inject my regular insulin to get the most consistent absorption?*

▼
TIP:

W e recommend that you use your abdomen. Insulin injected into the abdomen is absorbed quickly and predictably so you know how it will affect your blood sugar time after time. In general, there are three places to inject insulin—the abdomen, the arms, and the legs. Several factors affect the way your body absorbs insulin. If you exercise the muscles of your arms or legs vigorously after an injection, more insulin will be absorbed more quickly. It will be difficult for you to predict how this insulin will affect your blood sugar. Warm temperatures also increase the speed at which insulin is absorbed. Because your abdomen is usually covered by clothing and stays warm, insulin is absorbed more rapidly from this area.

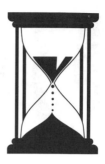

*H*ow long will my injection of regular insulin last?

▼
TIP:

Regular insulin generally lasts from 3 to 6 hours. However, the length of time that regular insulin lasts depends on the number of units that you inject. It also depends on how sensitive you are to insulin in your blood. The more regular insulin you inject, the longer its action lasts. One unit of insulin may last only 1 hour, whereas 10 units of insulin may last 5 hours or more. If you take a small dose of regular insulin before breakfast and your blood sugar starts to rise before lunch, you probably need to increase your regular insulin dose before breakfast. The same concept applies to lispro insulin, which generally lasts 2 to 3 hours. With normal doses of lispro insulin, your blood sugar will begin to rise after 4 hours unless you also take a background insulin such as NPH or ultralente.

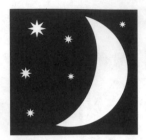

What can I do about low blood sugars at 3:00 A.M. if I take my last dose of regular and NPH insulin before supper?

▼
TIP:

An easy answer is to move your NPH injection to right before bedtime. You may also need to eat a late night snack before you go to bed. Another successful approach is to change to ultralente insulin. Human NPH insulin usually has a maximum effect 8–10 hours after you take it. If you take your insulin at dinnertime (6:00 P.M.), its peak of activity will be at about 4:00 A.M. Because you have also used up the food you ate at dinner by this time, you will probably have low blood sugar (hypoglycemia) at 3:00 A.M. When you have made adjustments to your regimen, get up at 3:00 A.M. and check your blood sugar level to be sure things are going as you planned.

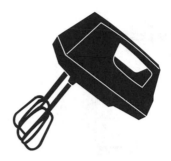

If I mix my regular insulin with my NPH or ultralente, will this reduce the effectiveness of my regular insulin?

▼
TIP:

No and yes. You can mix regular insulin with NPH insulin without altering the effect of your regular insulin. But, you cannot mix regular insulin with lente or ultralente insulin without risking some loss of the regular insulin's effect. The reason for this loss is that both lente and ultralente insulins contain excess zinc, which binds to the regular insulin and slows its absorption. If you do choose to mix regular and lente (or ultralente), you will need to inject it immediately after mixing up the dose, so the zinc does not have time to bind to the regular insulin. It is best to take separate injections (although inconvenient) if your schedule includes regular insulin plus one of the lente insulins.

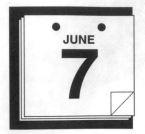

How often should I adjust the dose of my intermediate- or long-acting insulin if my blood sugar is not well-controlled?

▼
TIP:

Don't change your dose of intermediate- or long-acting insulin more often than every 3 or 4 days. Many factors besides insulin affect blood sugar levels. Some of these factors are exercise, how much food you eat, what you eat, illness, and the speed at which your injected insulin is absorbed. Until you have looked at these other factors, you should not adjust your intermediate- or long-acting insulin daily. Give your insulin schedule several days to work before trying a new one.

The same is true for regular or lispro insulin. You may make adjustments for a one-time high blood sugar, but changes to your regimen should come only after you've checked all the factors that affect your blood sugar level.

*H*ow can I get my blood sugars
under control when I have to
rotate between night and day shifts
on my job?

▼
TIP:

C learly, the best option is to negotiate with your employer to stay
on one shift. The Americans with Disabilities Act requires
employers to provide "reasonable accommodation for people with
diabetes." Or you may want to try a more flexible insulin regimen.
Using ultralente with regular insulin or an insulin pump will give
you the flexibility this situation demands. One of your problems is
that your body releases hormones during sleep that make insulin
work less effectively. By rotating shifts, you disturb the normal
release of these hormones. You don't know when the hormones are
being released, so you don't know how your insulin will affect your
blood sugar levels.

If I am using ultralente plus regular or lispro insulin, do I always need to take regular or lispro insulin at lunch even if I am not going to eat?

▼
TIP:

If your blood sugar is near normal, you probably don't need to take any additional insulin. If your blood sugar is high, you may want to take a "touch-up" dose of regular insulin at lunchtime even if you are not going to eat. Consider taking 1–5 units of regular insulin to bring your blood sugar back to normal before dinnertime. Taking an injection at lunchtime is almost always necessary if you are using lispro insulin because your breakfast injection will be almost completely gone by lunchtime. This is particularly true if you are taking only one injection of ultralente in the evening. If you are splitting your ultralente dose to twice a day (as we recommend), you may not need to take regular or lispro insulin at lunchtime if you do not eat lunch. With experience you will learn how much short-acting insulin to take.

*W*hat should I do if dinner is served and it has only been 15 minutes since I took my regular insulin?

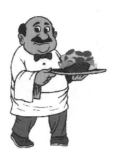

▼
TIP:

Foods that are high in carbohydrates (such as bread, starches, fruit, and milk) raise blood sugar rapidly. Protein foods may be partly converted to blood sugar, but the rise in blood sugar will be much later (after the meal). Ideally, you should wait 30–45 minutes before eating for regular insulin to start working. If this is not possible, try eating first the foods that won't have much effect on your blood sugar, such as the salad and meat, or sip on sugar-free drinks like iced tea. Save the starches, such as bread and potatoes, and eat them last so the regular insulin has another 10–15 minutes to work. In the future, you might consider changing to lispro insulin, which can be taken 0–15 minutes before the meal if your blood sugar is normal.

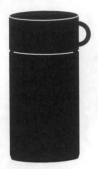

*H*ow should I store my insulin during a long car trip?

▼
TIP:

Your insulin is good at room temperature for at least 1 month. If you keep your insulin cooler than 85°F while traveling, it will be fine. If you are going to leave it in the car while you're out sightseeing, keep it in a small thermos and maybe even put the thermos in your ice chest. Don't put the bottle of insulin in direct contact with the ice in the cooler because freezing the insulin is just as bad as overheating it. If you are camping out in winter, keep your insulin bottle in your thermos or sleeping bag to prevent it from freezing.

*W*hat causes my regular insulin to get
cloudy after several weeks?

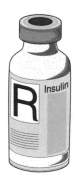

TIP:

A ll insulins have a tendency to change while they are stored.
Many factors speed up this change, including warm temperatures and shaking the insulin bottle. For this reason, you should not
carry your insulin in your pocket, especially if you are an active person. Keep it in your refrigerator, cupboard, purse, bricfcase, or back-
pack, and protect it from heat and motion. If regular insulin becomes
cloudy, throw it away. It has lost its effectiveness. It will not keep
your blood sugar from getting too high.

If you inject a mixture of regular and NPH or ultralente insulins,
you may be getting NPH or ultralcnte in the bottle of regular
insulin. This will make it cloudy, too. If in doubt, discard the old
bottle and replace it with a new bottle.

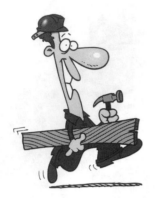

How can I take insulin at lunch when I'm on a constuction crew and can't be carrying insulin, syringes, or test supplies with me?

▼
TIP:

You could look at the blood glucose monitors and injection devices that are the size and shape of pocket pens. Because you can carry these instruments in your pocket, they provide a convenient way to monitor your sugar and inject the appropriate amount of insulin at work. Your diabetes health professional can provide you with information about these devices. Also, *Diabetes Forecast* magazine reviews the characteristics of these devices and others in the *Resource Guide*, which is published as a supplement to *Forecast* each December.

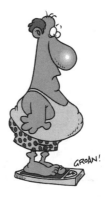

If I intentionally omit my insulin dose, will I lose weight?

▼
TIP:

Not really. Although recent studies have suggested that some patients do skip an insulin injection to lose weight, we don't recommend it. Skipping an injection is very hard on your system and docs not accomplish your goal of fat loss. Omitting an insulin injection lets your blood sugar rise, and you lose proteins, salts, and fluid in your urine. This can make you very ill, perhaps to the point of having to be hospitalized. Do not omit your insulin injection to lose weight.

Chapter 5
ORAL MEDICATION TIPS

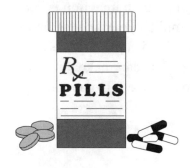

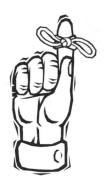

How can I remember to take my diabetes pills to prevent high blood sugars?

▼ TIP:

The best way to remember to take medication is to develop a daily routine. That is, always take the medication at the same time of day and in the same location, such as in the bathroom or at the breakfast table. To further reduce the chance of forgetting to take your medication, use a labeled pill box or pill organizer. These inexpensive boxes are available at drugstores. Set up medications in the pill box a week in advance to make it easy to know whether all your pills have been taken. The more medications you take, and the more complicated your pill-taking schedule is, the greater the likelihood that you will make mistakes. The danger of not taking diabetes medication is that your blood sugar levels will go very high.

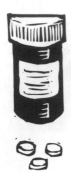

*W*hat should I do if I forget to take my diabetes
pills?

▼
TIP:

If you forget to take your oral diabetes medication, it is important
to know whether to take it when you do remember. The rule is
simple. If you are within 3 hours of the time of the dose you missed
(and you normally take pills twice per day), go ahead and take your
medication. If more than 3 hours have passed, wait for your next
scheduled dose. If you are on a long-acting medication that you take
once a day, take your medication if you are within 12 hours of miss-
ing your dose. Otherwise, wait until the next scheduled time to
resume taking your medication.

This plan is appropriate for medications in the classes of
sulfonylureas (such as Glucotrol), biguanides (such as Glucophage),
and thiazolidinedione (such as Rezulin). For medications such as
acarbose (Precose) or repaglinide (Prandin), wait until your next
meal to take these medications.

*W*hat do you suggest that I do
when my doctor wants me to
take insulin, but I would rather
take pills for my diabetes?

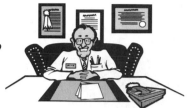

▼
TIP:

If you have type 1 diabetes, pills will not work for you. You will have to take insulin injections. However, if you have type 2 diabetes, then you may respond to pills. Many doctors try pills in patients with type 2 diabetes, because pills are easier to take and have other advantages. Tell your doctor that you would like to try the pills, and if they do not work, then you would be willing to take insulin injections. There is not an absolute "yes or no" blood test to tell how you will respond to pills. The only way to know is to try them for several weeks. Beginning to exercise (or increasing your level of physical activity) will help you gain better control with diabetes pills, too.

If you have type 2 diabetes and are taking insulin, you should talk to your doctor. Two new medications (metformin and troglitazone) have permitted some people with diabetes to switch to pills and stop their injections. Many new medications for diabetes are currently being tested, so stay in touch with your diabetes health care team.

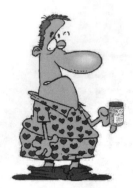

*W*hy does my doctor want me to take insulin at bedtime even though I am already taking pills for diabetes?

▼
TIP:

Your doctor is probably concerned about your fasting (before breakfast) blood sugar being high. When pills are not keeping your fasting blood sugar within the normal range, it is common practice to have you take insulin at night, so that your blood sugar is normal at the start of the day. You do much better with pills if your blood sugar level before breakfast is in the normal range. If this program does not work for you, you may have to take insulin both in the morning and at night, even though you have type 2 diabetes.

Chapter 6
SICK DAY TIPS

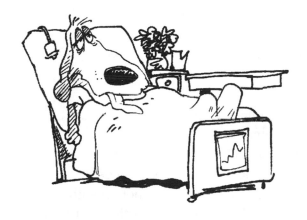

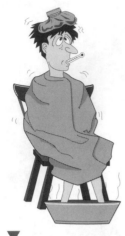

*W**hen I am ill with the flu, what should I do to keep my blood sugar from going too high?***

▼
TIP:

Monitor three factors every 4 hours when you are sick:

1. Your blood sugar
2. Your urine ketones
3. Your body weight

High blood sugar indicates that you need more regular insulin. High urine ketones indicate that your body needs more carbohydrate intake (sugar-containing drinks and more insulin) to suppress fat breakdown. A loss of weight indicates that you need more fluids. When you cannot get your blood sugar below 250 mg/dl, your urine ketones below 3+, or your body weight close to normal, then you must call your health care team.

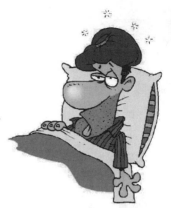

When I am sick with the flu and cannot eat food without vomiting, how do I know how much insulin to take?

▼

TIP:

The guide to how much insulin to take is your current blood sugar. You need to take enough regular insulin to keep your blood sugar below 200 mg/dl, so that you do not become dehydrated due to excessive urination. For adults, we recommend taking an injection of at least 5 units of regular insulin every 4 hours and to keep increasing the dose of regular insulin by 1 unit until your blood sugar gets below 200 mg/dl. This may be more than your usual dose of insulin even though you are not eating. If you inject regular insulin every 4 hours, you should probably withhold your intermediate- or long-acting insulin until you get well. (Check with your health care provider.) Of course, if you are relying solely on regular insulin, you will need to wake up during the night to take an insulin injection. If you are taking lispro insulin, the dose of the insulin is the same but you must continue your background intermediate- or long-acting insulin.

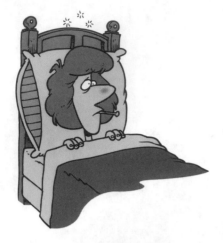

Will fever increase my blood sugar and, therefore, my need for insulin?

▼
TIP:

Yes. Even mild illness may require you to take a little more insulin. And if you develop a fever with chills, muscle aches, and sweating, you will definitely need increasing doses of insulin. In fact, your requirements of regular or lispro insulin may double. Keep a thermometer at home to determine when your body temperature is above 99°F, because this and frequent blood sugar checks are the keys to knowing when you need more insulin. You and your health care team should develop a plan for what to do if your blood sugar is high when you are sick. Do not hesitate to call them when you are ill.

*A*t what point must I seek medical
help if I have the flu?

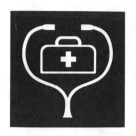

▼
TIP:

You should seek medical help when you cannot keep down liquids. Contrary to popular belief, eating solid food is not essential during short-term illness. Most people have ample body fat stores to provide energy. However, you must be able to drink liquids and, preferably, carbohydrate-containing fluids. If you are unable to hold down any fluids for more than 12 hours, you need to seek medical help immediately. Your body will become dehydrated if you can't ingest salt and water. This can affect you seriously, causing acidosis, unconsciousness, and death. Therefore, if you are vomiting all fluids or are spilling large amounts of ketones in your urine, you should contact your health care team immediately.

Ideally, you should set up a sick-day plan with your health care team before you ever get sick. That way you will have more information about who to call and when.

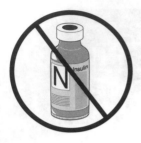

Should I skip my NPH insulin dose in the morning before a dental appointment that prevents me from eating lunch?

▼
TIP:

Not necessarily. You have two options. The first option is to omit the A.M. dose of NPH but take your regular or lispro insulin dose before you eat breakfast. You must take a dose of regular or lispro insulin about 5–6 hours after your morning dose of regular insulin (this second small dose is to keep your blood sugar under control even though you won't be eating).

The second option is to take your regular or lispro insulin and then to cut your morning NPH dose by about 1/3 (because you won't be eating lunch) and inject that. After the dental procedure (about 6 hours after your a.m. dose of regular or lispro insulin), check your blood sugar, and if necessary, you can take an additional small dose of regular or lispro insulin that should tide you over until dinnertime.

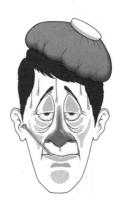

Why are my sugars still high when I had the flu a week ago?

▼
TIP:

Major stresses cause changes in the body that may last for several weeks beyond the time when you get well. Although you may feel better now, these changes (which affect many of the substances in your body that raise blood sugar) are still active. Remember that you may need additional insulin for 1–2 weeks after a major stress (for example, severe flu, surgery, pneumonia, or heart attack) to keep your blood sugar levels in the normal range.

Chapter 7
NUTRITION TIPS

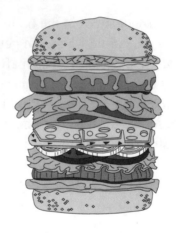

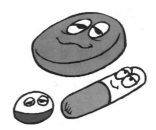

Should I take vitamins or minerals to improve my blood sugar?

▼
TIP:

There is not enough scientific evidence to recommend vitamin or mineral supplements to improve your blood sugar. From time to time, various vitamin and mineral supplements have been popular. Recently, magnesium, chromium, zinc, vanadium, and selenium have been publicized by the media and promoted by health food stores as having a beneficial effect on blood sugar. Nevertheless, eating foods that contain the vitamins and minerals, such as fruits and vegetables, is still the best way to get what your body needs.

In contrast, we strongly recommend that you get pneumonia vaccinations (available all year) and annual flu vaccinations (available in early fall). Vaccinations may prevent (or reduce the severity of) these illnesses, which usually cause high blood sugars. Ask your health care team for their advice.

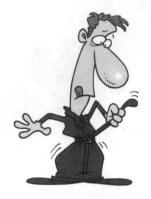

*H*ow can I lose weight when I
hardly eat anything now?

▼
TIP:

If you are not exercising, you will be surprised at the difference a
daily 30-minute walk can make in both weight loss and blood
sugar control. Walking burns calories and lowers blood sugar. If
exercise becomes a daily habit, you'll need to adjust the amount of
insulin you take and the food you eat.

Another way to lose weight may be as simple as reducing the
food you eat by one slice of bread per day. One slice of bread
contains 80–100 calories, and 30 slices of bread (amount eaten in 1
month) is equal to approximately 1 pound of body weight.
Therefore, if you omit one of your usual slices of bread per day for
1 year, you may possibly lose up to 12 pounds!

Keep a journal of the foods you eat for 3–5 days. Also record
when you eat and the emotion or situation that preceded eating.
Most people are surprised to find that they do eat more than they
realize, or that certain situations always trigger overeating. Your
ability to keep a food diary and learn from it will help you lose
weight.

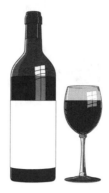

*H*ow will alcohol affect my blood sugar?

▼
TIP:

A lcohol interferes with your body's ability to produce blood sugar and causes low blood sugar. Do not drink alcohol if you are not eating. If you are eating a meal and you drink only a small quantity of alcohol, then the alcohol should not cause you to have a severe problem with low blood sugar. You will, however, need to include the calories that are in the alcohol in your meal plan. In general, one alcoholic beverage substitutes for 1 fat exchange in a meal plan. Check with your registered dietitian (RD) for help with this.

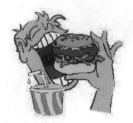

How can I lose weight and keep eating the foods that I like?

▼
TIP:

You do not have to give up all the foods that you like. It's the size of the portion you eat that is important. Some foods are higher in fat content than other foods. If you cut down on or cut out high-fat foods altogether, you can lose significant amounts of weight. To find the fat and caloric content of the foods you eat, look for paperback books that list this information. These books can be found at libraries, bookstores, and pharmacies. See how much fat is in your favorite foods. Eliminating even one high-fat food that you eat often will result in weight loss. Remember that exercise will make it even easier to lose weight.

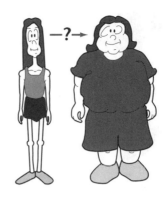

Will I gain weight as I lower my blood sugar?

▼
TIP:

Not necessarily, especially if you keep track of how much you eat. However, many people do gain weight, and the reasons are complex. One factor is that you are no longer losing large quantities of calories in your urine (in the form of glucose). An equal number of calories (equal to what was being lost in your urine) will need to be deleted from the amount of food you eat. You won't know how many calories this is unless you monitor your weight and what you eat. If you start to gain weight, reduce the amount of food you eat and exercise more. If lowering your blood sugar causes you to have more low blood sugar reactions, then the food that you eat to treat the reactions may add to a weight gain.

W*hy don't some sugar-free foods taste very good?*

▼ TIP:

While some foods are actually improved by becoming sugar free (canned fruit, for example), other foods are not so successfully converted to sugar free. These are usually foods in which artificial sweeteners (sorbitol, saccharin, or aspartame) are added to taste sweet. But these sweeteners do not cook like sugar, so they don't work well in baked foods and may leave a bitter aftertaste. Also, remember that these foods are not necessarily low in calories. For example, sugar-free pudding made with reduced-fat milk has 90 calories per serving as compared to 140 calories per serving for regular pudding. Although 90 is less than 140, it still isn't calorie free. You don't have to eat only sugar-free cookies. You may have a real cookie—just include it in your meal plan.

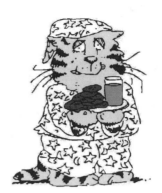

*H*ow *large a snack should I eat at bedtime?*

▼
TIP:

You should eat about 1/7 of your total calories per day before you go to sleep if you have a normal blood sugar level. Your bedtime snack is designed to keep enough glucose in your blood so that your blood sugar does not get too low in the middle of the night. The NPH or ultralente insulin you took before supper can peak during this time and cause low blood sugar. Your health care provider or RD can help you adjust your snack to work with your insulin or medication dose, so that your morning blood sugar will be in the normal range.

A snack may not be necessary if your bedtime blood sugar is above 180 mg/dl. If your bedtime blood sugar is lower than 180 mg/dl, you will probably want to have a snack that includes starch and protein, such as peanut butter and crackers or low-fat cheese on toast. You may need to add a glass of fat-free milk or a serving of fruit if your blood sugar is less than 100 mg/dl.

BEDTIME SNACK SUMMARY

Blood Sugar (mg/dl)	Snack Quantity
<100	juice or milk and usual snack
101–180	usual snack
>181	no snack

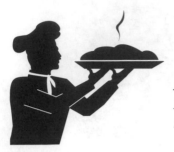

My goal is to be normal weight with near normal blood sugars, so how do I reduce fat in a meal when I eat at a restaurant?

▼
TIP:

Meat is the best place to start cutting fat calories. If you order fish that is broiled or baked, it will usually have less than 5 grams of fat per ounce. If you order a meat serving from the menu, look for foods that are grilled or broiled. Also look for a lower-fat meat, such as sirloin, instead of prime rib or filet. Ask the waiter how many ounces are in the serving size. You may even be able to request a particular serving size, such as "only a 4-ounce serving of the sirloin" or request that the meat be prepared with no fat. Other sources of fat are gravies and sauces. You can request that the sauce be served on the side, and check it out before you find your chicken breast swimming in butter. Meats that are processed, such as bratwurst, lunch meats, and sausages, can be very high in fat (as much as 10–15 grams per ounce) and are usually very high in salt as well.

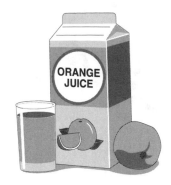

*H*ow can I have orange juice for breakfast without risking high blood sugars later?

▼
TIP:

It is better for you to eat the orange (or any other fruit) than to drink the juice from that fruit. If you like the bright wake-up taste of orange juice first thing in the morning, you might try mixing 1/2 juice and 1/2 water. Or you could try a sugar-free citrus-flavored drink mix (and a serving of real fruit later in the day). You will get the tangy orange taste without any sugar! It isn't so much the sugar in the orange but the liquid form that makes orange juice (or any other juice) raise your blood sugar rapidly. Studies comparing juice and sugar-containing soft drinks found that there is no difference in the effect they have on people's blood sugar. We advise people to use juice as "treatment" for low blood sugar, not as food.

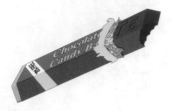

Can I eat candy bars now that the ADA is including table sugar in meal plans?

▼
TIP:

Sometimes. It is true that the most recent dietary guidelines for people with diabetes include simple sugars, including table sugar. Several studies have shown that table sugar eaten as part of a meal plan does not have any worse effect on blood glucose than rice or potatoes. This does not mean, however, that people with diabetes can eat sweets freely. Sugars must be included as part of your meal plan. And the reason you still want to limit the number of candy bars you eat is that most of the calories in candy bars come from fat. Fat should be limited in everybody's diet! Also, the calories in candy bars are "empty" calories—that is, they don't give you the vitamins or minerals that you need to be healthy.

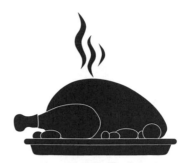

How can I keep my blood sugar normal during the holidays when high-calorie, high-fat foods are served?

▼
TIP:

Holidays are always difficult because of the change in daily routine and the increased availability of high-calorie, high-fat foods. We recommend several approaches to preventing your hemoglobin A1c from rising during the holidays.

First, a week before the holiday, try to control your blood sugars, so that any indulgences during the holiday will be balanced by these better than usual blood sugar levels.

Second, make it a point never to eat between scheduled meals, even if cakes and cookies are available. Sticking to standard mealtimes will keep your diabetes medications on schedule and prevent high blood sugars.

Third, never accept second portions at any meal, even though they are offered. Simply tell your host that you are full. Don't let the holidays disturb your blood sugar control, and you'll feel better during and after the festivities.

Fourth, exercise more. Take a walk!

Fifth, if you do eat more than usual, adjust your insulin upward.

Chapter 8
EXERCISE TIPS

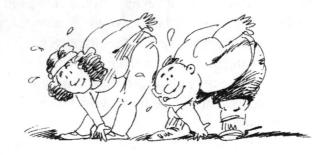

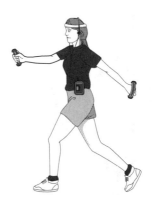

How can I get the regular exercise that I need to improve my blood sugar?

▼
TIP:

Walk. Many people are surprised to learn that walking is an excellent exercise. We recommend walking for everyone. You burn approximately 200 calories in a 1-hour walk. You will lose 1 pound every 2 1/2 weeks from this 1 hour of exercise (providing that you don't increase the amount of food you eat). Walk to the shopping center, the supermarket, or the corner drugstore instead of driving. Walking is easy on the muscles and joints and rarely causes low blood sugar. Exercise may make your body more sensitive to insulin, so it can help you achieve a normal body weight and a normal blood sugar level. Start walking today!

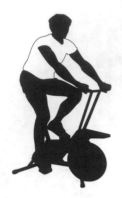

*D*oes exercise raise or lower my blood sugar?

▼
TIP:

Exercise will either raise or lower your blood sugar depending on how much insulin is in your blood. Muscles use glucose, so your blood sugar level gets lower during exercise. This level will go even lower if there is a lot of insulin in your blood. But you must have some insulin circulating in your blood or, in response to exercise, your liver will make more glucose, causing your blood sugar level to rise.

Check your blood sugar before you exercise. If it is low, you can drink a sugar-containing beverage. If it is high, you can take a small dose of regular (or lispro) insulin. If it is higher than 300 mg/dl, we recommend that you delay exercise until the insulin you have taken lowers your glucose to less than 250 mg/dl. The more intense the exercise, the more difficult it is to predict whether your blood sugar will increase or decrease. If you exercise for a long time, recheck your blood sugar halfway through. With experience, you will be able to predict how your exercise will affect your blood sugar levels. You may notice a blood sugar–lowering effect for as long as 24 hours after heavy exercise.

*H*ow much food do I need to eat to avoid low blood sugars when I exercise?

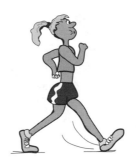

▼
TIP:

The amount of food needed to prevent low blood sugar during or after exercise is different for each person. In general, if your blood sugar is below 150 mg/dl before exercising, having a snack of 15 grams of carbohydrate is a good idea (one serving of starch, fruit, or milk). If you have problems with low blood sugars much later after exercise, have a snack of 15–30 grams of carbohydrate within 30 minutes of finishing the exercise to help your body replace the glucose normally stored in muscle and to prevent low blood sugar later. This could be a sandwich, 5–10 saltine crackers, or 4–8 vanilla wafers or animal cookies. If you are exercising immediately before or after a meal, you may be able to reduce the regular insulin used for meal coverage, because the exercise will reduce your blood sugar, which normally increases following a meal.

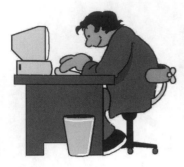

Why do I get low blood sugar when I mow the lawn on Saturday morning but never when I'm at my desk during the week?

▼
TIP:

Muscles use blood glucose to do work, so if you eat the same amount of food and take the same dose of insulin, you can expect your blood sugar to be lower on the day when you are more physically active. You have four choices:

1. Eat more carbohydrate with breakfast.
2. Decrease your morning dose of Regular insulin (about 20–40% less is usually needed to allow for an hour of yard work).
3. Eat a mid-morning snack to prevent the hypoglycemia.
4. Let your grass grow.

*W*hy does my blood sugar get low in the middle of the night after I exercise during the day?

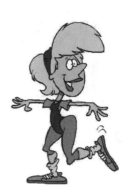

▼
TIP:

E xercise is good for you, but it can bring on low blood sugar in several ways. Exercise helps you use insulin more efficiently so that a given amount of insulin has more blood sugar–lowering power. These effects of exercise can last for up to 24 hours after the exercise has ended. That's why insulin doses should usually be decreased before and after exercise. Also, you should eat a meal or have a snack before exercising if your blood sugar is normal or low. If you balance your insulin, your food intake, and your exercise, you will have fewer low blood sugars during the night after your daytime exercise.

Why do I always seem to get low blood sugar after having sex?

▼
TIP:

S ex is just as much an exercise as jogging or aerobics. Planning to eat food either immediately before or shortly after sex to cover the glucose that you use is the way to avoid low blood sugar. You may want to check your blood sugar first, even though it may reduce the spontaneity of the moment. You might also consider increasing your snack before going to bed.

Chapter 9
EDUCATIONAL TIPS

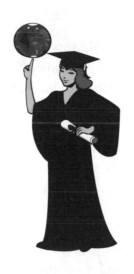

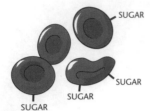

*W*hat is the *"glycosylated hemoglobin test"?*

▼
TIP:

The glycosylated hemoglobin test measures the percentage of hemoglobin molecules (the chemical in our blood that carries oxygen) that have sugar attached to them. Because this percentage directly reflects the average blood sugar levels over the life of a red blood cell (90 days), this information helps you and your health care team assess your overall blood sugar control. There are several different tests that are used to measure glycosylated hemoglobin (such as a test called hemoglobin A_{1c}), and each test has its own normal range and target values. Ask your doctor what test s/he is using and what the target value should be for you. The glycosylated hemoglobin test, along with self-monitoring of blood sugar, has made good blood sugar control possible for people with diabetes.

*W*here can I find new
information that will help me
with my blood sugar management?

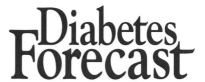

▼
TIP:

There are several ways to find out about new discoveries and products that will help you control your blood sugar levels. You can call the ADA's national center (800) DIABETES [(800) 342-2383] to ask for information. Or you can call (888) DIABETES, and you will be connected to the ADA office nearest you. They may have information about new products and techniques to treat diabetes. You can subscribe to *Diabetes Forecast*, a magazine for people with diabetes published by the ADA. This magazine has many articles that help you keep up to date. ADA has other books and publications about diabetes that you can buy in bookstores or order over the phone by calling (800) 232-6733. Many health professionals, such as nurses and RDs, specialize in diabetes care and are called certified diabetes educators or CDEs. They have a wealth of information about diabetes. Ask your doctor to recommend a diabetes educator to help you manage your diabetes. For a list of CDEs in your area, call the ADA at (800) DIABETES or the American Association of Diabetes Educators (AADE) at (800) TEAM-UP-4 [(800) 832-6874].

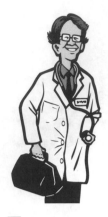

Should I see a diabetes specialist for my diabetes care?

TIP:

In the U.S., 80% of people with diabetes see physicians who are family practice or general practice physicians. If you feel you are getting your blood sugar levels into the goal range and have a good relationship with your doctor, you do not need a diabetes specialist. Sometimes your family doctor will refer you to a specialist for occasional visits or a consultation to get some help with managing your diabetes, but then you can continue your routine care with your family physician. If your primary care doctor can't help you with the daily activities of living with diabetes, you may benefit from diabetes education. Call ADA at (800) DIABETES or AADE at (800) TEAM-UP-4 [(800) 832-6874] to locate a diabetes educator or diabetes education program in your area.

*H*ow often should I see my
doctor to keep my blood sugar
under control?

CALENDAR			
JANUARY	FEBRUARY ✔	MARCH	APRIL
MAY ✔	JUNE	JULY	AUGUST ✔
SEPTEMBER	OCTOBER	NOVEMBER ✔	DECEMBER

▼
TIP:

*A*s you tighten control of your diabetes, you will need to see your
doctor weekly or every 2 weeks, at first. How often you see
your doctor, RD, or diabetes educator will depend on how long you
have had diabetes, your ability to adjust your medication for tight
blood sugar control, and whether you have any diabetic complications or other medical problems that may interfere with your diabetes management. After that, a visit every 3 months may be enough
to reach your target goals.

At a minimum, you should plan on seeing your doctor twice a
year to arrange for necessary eye and kidney checkups and to stay
motivated about good blood sugar control. You should have someone
you can contact on short notice to discuss problems as they arise,
such as unexplained high blood sugars or sudden illness. This person
does not have to be a physician but may be a CDE, RD, nurse practi-
tioner, or nurse case manager.

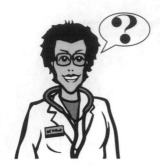

Why does my doctor ask me about the average blood sugar reading on my monitor?

▼
TIP:

You can use the average blood sugar that your meter calculates to improve your blood sugar control. These averages are not a true average of your blood sugar levels but only an average of the times you've actually tested. (If, like most people with diabetes, you measure your blood sugar before meals and at bedtime, this value could more accurately be called your average premeal blood sugar.) People with diabetes with good blood sugar control maintain this average blood sugar below 120 mg/dl. If your average is much higher than this, then you know that you need to adjust your diabetes management program.

*H*ow *does the glycosylated
hemoglobin or hemoglobin
A_{1c} (HbA$_{1c}$) help me monitor
my blood sugar control?*

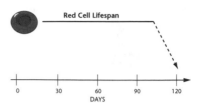

▼
TIP:

These tests tell you how well you are controlling your blood
sugar over a period of several months. Glycosylated hemoglobin
and hemoglobin A_{1c} are names for tests that measure how much glucose (blood sugar) is attached to your red blood cells. This interac-
tion with glucose occurs slowly and becomes permanent over time.
Because a red blood cell stays in your body 120 days, measuring
how much glucose is attached to your red blood cells is a good indi-
cation of your average blood sugar over a 2- to 4-month period. It
cannot, however, tell whether you are having frequent ups and
downs in your blood sugar levels. Studies have shown that the lower
your glycosylated hemoglobin or hemoglobin A_{1c}, the less likely
you are to have many of the complications caused by diabetes.

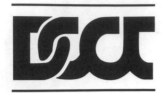

What is the DCCT and how does it affect me?

▼
TIP:

The DCCT is the Diabetes Control and Complications Trial, a long-term diabetes study that proved the complications of diabetes can be delayed or prevented by good blood sugar control. More than 1,400 people with type 1 diabetes were enrolled in this study at centers all across America for a period of 5–8 years. Half of these people received "conventional" diabetes care (1–2 insulin injections per day), and half received "intensive" diabetes management (as many injections as necessary to maintain near-normal blood sugar). People in the intensive therapy group had significantly fewer diabetic complications. As a result of the DCCT, everyone with diabetes (type 1 or 2) should be working to keep his or her blood sugar levels close to normal.

Intensive Therapy Group of the DCCT

Diabetic eye disease	76% decreased risk
Diabetic kidney disease	54% decreased risk
Diabetic nerve disease	60% decreased risk

*H*ow does the health of my teeth affect my blood sugar control?

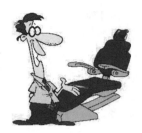

▼
TIP:

Chronic gum disease can be a cause of unexplained high blood sugars. People with diabetes should have their teeth professionally cleaned at least twice a year because they have a much higher risk of developing gum disease than people without diabetes. Gum disease results from the formation of plaque underneath the gum line after eating. Plaque hardens into tartar, which irritates the gums and gradually erodes the underlying bone that holds the teeth in place. Thus, gum disease can lead to the need for dentures. Daily dental care can prevent gum disease from getting started. Brush your teeth at least twice a day with a soft bristle brush and floss daily. Flossing removes food from between the teeth and plaque from the gum line.

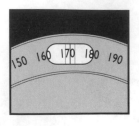

Why have I gained 15 pounds over the 3 years that I have been working to improve my blood sugar control?

TIP:

Some people who practice "intensified management" to keep their diabetes under control gain weight. Because insulin is a hormone that helps your body process the food you eat, one of its many actions is to store fat. It makes sense, then, that injecting insulin to keep your blood sugar down will also result in increased fat storage. The reasons you want good blood sugar control (for example, to decrease your risk of eye and kidney disease) are usually more important than this potential weight gain. The best way to avoid gaining weight is to develop an active lifestyle and follow your health care team's recommended meal plan, limiting fat and total calories.

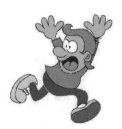

*H*ow can I encourage my child to take
insulin injections if he or she is
scared to death of needles?

▼
TIP:

Try one of the insulin injection devices on the market that do not use needles. They inject insulin by squirting it into the skin at high pressure. Some people with "needle phobia" prefer this method of insulin delivery. Blood sugar control with these devices is as good or better than that achieved with syringe-injected insulin. Although cumbersome and expensive, one of these devices used for a few weeks or months may help your child to become more comfortable with the process so that s/he will be willing to try using the syringe to inject the insulin.

See the tip on inhaled insulin on page 120. You may need to see a mental health professional with your child to help both of you get past this difficulty.

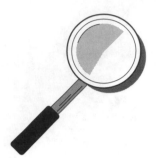

My eyesight is very poor—how can I read the numbers on my glucose meter and then correctly fill my syringe?

▼
TIP:

Many people with diabetes have visual problems. For this reason, there are blood glucose meters that also announce your results. You will be able to check the numbers you can see against the numbers you can hear. To read the numbers on your insulin syringe, you can use a magnifying glass or buy a magnifier that fits on the syringe. You might also consider using a pen-like insulin injector that gives a specific amount of insulin with each click, which you hear as you turn the dial or push the plunger. Your doctor or ADA can provide you with information on both of these devices.

Chapter 10
NEW TIPS

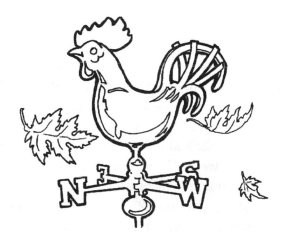

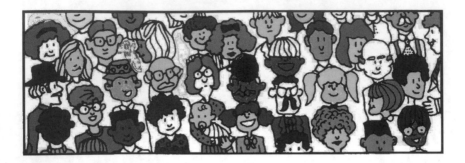

W*hat is the "UKPDS" study?*

▼
TIP:

UKPDS stands for United Kingdom Prospective Diabetes Study, the longest and largest study in patients with type 2 diabetes that has ever been performed. More than 5,000 patients with newly diagnosed type 2 diabetes were studied in 21 different centers in the United Kingdom between 1977 and 1991. This study showed that eye disease, kidney disease, and possibly nerve disease were preventable as a result of lowering blood glucose levels with intensive therapy. It also demonstrated that for every percentage point decrease in hemoglobin A_{1c} (from 9% down to 8%), there was a 25% reduction in diabetes-related deaths. It also demonstrated that lowering blood pressure in people with type 2 diabetes to an average of at least 144/82 mmHg significantly reduced strokes, diabetes-related deaths, heart failure, microvascular (small blood vessel) complications, and loss of vision. This study's results were similar to the DCCT results for people with type 1 diabetes. It emphasizes how important it is for people with type 2 diabetes to bring their blood pressure and blood glucose close to normal levels.

Does smoking affect my glucose control?

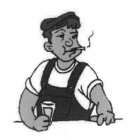

▼
TIP:

Yes. Studies have demonstrated that people who smoke have an increased resistance to insulin. This means that whatever insulin you take (or whatever insulin is secreted by your pancreas) does not work as well. Thus, getting your blood glucose close to normal is much more difficult. There are actually many reasons that people with diabetes should not smoke. The primary reason is that smoking is definitely a risk factor for heart disease. People with diabetes already have one strike against them as far as heart disease is concerned. Smoking also has many detrimental health effects, such as causing cancer, lung disease, and early aging. It would be wise to quit.

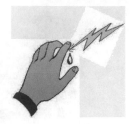

Is there a better way than using lancets to get blood from my finger for home blood glucose monitoring?

▼
TIP:

Yes. Although there is not yet a glucose meter available that will allow you to measure your blood sugar without drawing blood, there have been other advances in the field. Specifically, one company has developed a skin perforator that draws a drop of blood from your finger using a low-power laser beam. This device, called the Lasette, produces a small hole in your skin by vaporizing the outer layers of skin with a brief burst of energy. Studies have shown that this works as well as a stainless steel lancet. More important, most patients with diabetes who used the Lasette felt no pain, and 54% of the patients preferred the Lasette over the lancet. Use of the Lasette reduces medical waste and may reduce the risk of exposure to blood-borne diseases, such as Hepatitis B, which can be transmitted through a contaminated puncture wound. The Lasette has been approved for home use by the FDA, but whether or not you should purchase one depends on how much they cost, how often you sample your blood sugar, and how comfortable you are using the stainless steel lancets.

What should I expect from my child's school or day care regarding his or her diabetes care?

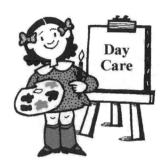

▼
TIP:

The responsibilities for diabetes care should be shared. You provide 1) a treatment plan, 2) all diabetes materials, 3) hypoglycemic treatment foods and snacks, and 4) emergency phone numbers.

The school or day-care center provides 1) immediate treatment for hypoglycemia, 2) an adult to check blood sugar and administer glucagon or insulin, 3) a private area for testing and insulin administration, 4) an adult to oversee the child's meal schedule, 5) access to school medical personnel, 6) permission to eat a snack whenever necessary, 7) permission to miss school for diabetes care with a note from the health care provider, 8) access to the bathroom and drinking water, and 9) storage for diabetes supplies.

The child is expected to 1) cooperate with diabetes tasks [age 8 or older], 2) perform blood glucose testing [7th grade and above], and 3) administer his/her own insulin [high school]. Finally, all children are expected to ask for help whenever necessary.

Discuss these points with the day-care center or school before enrolling your child.

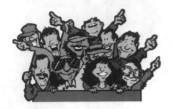

*W*ho should be screened for diabetes?

▼
TIP:

All people above the age of 45 should have a fasting morning blood sugar level test to see if they have diabetes. A fasting morning blood sugar level higher than 126 mg/dl on two occasions indicates diabetes. If they do not have diabetes, then the test should be repeated every 3 years. People who have specific risk factors for diabetes, even though they are younger than age 45, should probably be tested once a year. Such people include

1. individuals who weigh more than 120% of their ideal body weight
2. people with a parent or sibling who has diabetes
3. members of certain high-risk ethnic groups (African, Hispanic, and American Indians)
4. women who have delivered a baby weighing more than 9 pounds or who had gestational diabetes during a previous pregnancy
5. people with very low levels of HDL cholesterol (less than 35 mg/dl) or very high triglyceride levels (above 250 mg/dl)
6. people who have previously been diagnosed with impaired glucose tolerance (a prediabetic condition)

It is hoped that increased screening for diabetes will allow diagnosis at an earlier stage and so prevent the complications of the disease.

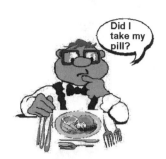

Will the new medication Prandin help my diabetes?

▼
TIP:

That depends on the type of diabetes you have and what your current diabetes therapy is. Prandin (repaglinide) stimulates your pancreas to produce insulin, much as sulfonylureas do. However, repaglinide is not a sulfonylurea and is not related structurally to any other medications currently on the market. The advantage of Prandin is that it works very quickly, so that it is taken with meals or up to 30 minutes prior to meals and reaches its peak effectiveness within 1 hour. It is gone from your bloodstream within 3 to 4 hours. Its primary action is to raise circulating insulin levels, primarily after meals, when glucose levels are high. Prandin can be used alone or in combination with some diabetes medications such as metformin (Glucophage). Side effects of Prandin are similar to those that occur with sulfonylurea treatment, such as weight gain and an occasional low blood sugar. However, it is generally safe in people who are elderly and people who have mild kidney and liver problems. The drawback of Prandin is the need to take it with each meal and, perhaps, the cost. If you would like to try this medication, discuss it with your health care team.

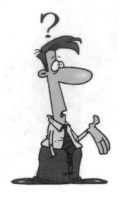

What is the best way to lower my blood sugar if my glyburide isn't working anymore?

▼
TIP:

Glyburide (Micronase, Diabeta) and related medicines like glipizide (Glucotrol) and glimepiride (Amaryl) belong to a class of drugs called sulfonylureas that work by causing your pancreas to release insulin. These medicines commonly lose their effectiveness after several years. In the past, adding insulin or switching to insulin were your only options. Currently, however, there are a number of other options, including adding a medication such as metformin (Glucophage), troglitazone (Rezulin), or acarbose (Precose) to the medicine you are already taking. Because these new medicines work differently from sulfonylureas, they often result in additional blood sugar lowering. All of these drugs reduce glycosylated hemoglobin by 1–2% when they are added to a sulfonylurea. Talk to your diabetes care team about the pros and cons of adding an additional diabetes medicine to your schedule, and try one for 3–6 months to see whether it works for you.

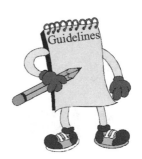

Should I be concerned with glucose control if I have type 2 diabetes?

▼
TIP:

Yes, but maybe not "tight" control. The older you were when you got diabetes, the less benefit you will get from achieving excellent glucose control. This change in benefit level means that your individual risk needs to be refigured before you decide what your target hemoglobin A_{1c} should be. The Veterans' Health Administration (VA) has developed guidelines that you can use depending on the age at which you developed type 2 diabetes. These guidelines are now used in all VA clinics. A patient with type 2 diabetes who developed diabetes at an elderly age may have a target hemoglobin A_{1c} of about 9%, whereas younger patients may benefit from a lower hemoglobin A_{1c} of 7%. If you would like details of these guidelines and what your target hemoglobin A_{1c} should probably be, you can obtain them on the Internet at http://www.va.gov/health/diabetes/default.htm (in the Management of Diabetes Mellitus Glycemic Control Annotations, Module G, Section G) or ask your health provider for information on this subject.

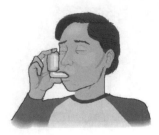

*C*an I inhale insulin, so that I no longer
have to take insulin shots?

▼
TIP:

If all goes well, you can expect to see inhaled insulin available to
you within the next 2 to 5 years. Powdered insulin is inhaled
through the mouth and absorbed by the lungs, using an inhaler similar to the device used by patients with asthma. The insulin that is
inhaled is very rapidly absorbed into the body. Inhaled insulin is
taken before each meal, and intermediate-acting insulin is injected at
bedtime. In one recent study in people with type 1 diabetes, 70 individuals used the inhaler and did as well as people taking insulin
injections. In patients with type 2 diabetes, a similar result was
observed in a study involving 51 participants. Additional studies are
planned, and if successful, the results will be submitted to the FDA
for approval. This type of insulin administration may be particularly
advantageous for children and anyone else who dislikes insulin
injections.

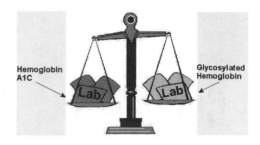

Hemoglobin
A1C

Glycosylated
Hemoglobin

What is the difference between glycosylated hemoglobin and hemoglobin A_{1c}?

▼
TIP:

These are both laboratory tests to measure how much sugar is stuck to the red blood cells that carry oxygen in your blood. Health care providers use these tests to estimate the level of diabetes control during the prior 3 months. Unfortunately, people often use the two terms interchangeably. There are several different kinds of hemoglobin in human red blood cells, and the glycosylated hemoglobin test measures how much sugar is stuck to all of them. The hemoglobin A_{1c} test, on the other hand, measures only how much sugar is stuck to a particular kind of hemoglobin—hemoglobin A_1. Both tests are accurate and reliable, but the normal levels differ, with hemoglobin A_{1c} levels typically being about 2% lower than total glycosylated hemoglobin levels. When your diabetes care team orders a glycosylated hemoglobin or hemoglobin A_{1c} test for you, ask for the normal (nondiabetic) levels so that you can interpret the test. In general, you should aim to keep your lycosylated hemoglobin or hemoglobin A_{1c} level close to the high end of the normal level. Ask your doctor about your level of glycosylated hemoglobin.

Chapter 11
RESOURCES

American Association of Diabetes Educators . . . .(800) 338-3633
    444 N. Michigan Ave. . . . .(312) 644-2233
    Suite 1240
    Chicago, IL 60611-3901

American Diabetes Association . . . .(800) 232-3472
    1660 Duke Street . . . .(703) 549-1500
    Alexandria, VA 22314

The American Dietetic Association . . . .(800) 366-1655
    216 West Jackson Blvd.
    Suite 800
    Chicago, IL 60606-6995

International Diabetic Athletes Association . . . .(800) 898-4322
    1647 W. Bethany Home Road, #B
    Phoenix, AZ 85015

National Diabetes Information Clearinghouse . . . . . .(301) 468-2162
    Box NDIC
    9000 Rockville Pike
    Bethesda, MD 20892

INDEX

A

Abdomen, insulin injections in, 55–56
Absorption, of insulin, 55–56
ACE inhibitors, 13
Adrenalin, 50
African, 116
Age factors, 19, 46, 113
Alcohol (beverage), 83
Alcohol (rubbing), sterilizing skin, 11
Altitude, glucose meter readings and, 52
American Association of Diabetes Educators, 101–102
American Diabetes Association, 5, 101
American Indians, 116
Americans with Disabilities Act, 61
Amputations, 26
Arms, insulin injections in, 55
Arterial hardening, 9
Artificial sweeteners, 86
Aspartame, 86
Average blood sugar levels, 4, 6, 17, 27, 104

B

Bedtime snacks, 41, 87, 98
Blindness, 26
Blood pressure, 112
  excess weight and, 18
  medication for, 13
  records of, 6
Blood sugar levels
  age and, 19, 46
  average, 4, 6, 17, 27, 104, 121
  blood pressure and, 13, 18, 112
  complications and, 9, 17, 19, 103, 106, 112–113
  elderly people, 19, 46
  excess weight and, 18
  exercise and. See Exercise
  eye disease and, 10, 112
  fasting, 72, 116
  goals for, 3, 5, 119, 121
  hemoglobin and. See Hemoglobin
  high. See Hyperglycemia
  improving, 8–9
  insulin pumps and, 15, 61
  intensified control of. See Intensified diabetes management
  job shift changes and, 61
  low. See Hypoglycemia
  meters for. See Meters, blood glucose
  monitoring, 20, 27–28, 35, 37, 40, 50, 66, 104–105, 114
  prediabetes, 4
  records of, 6
  sickness and. See Sickness
  slow digestion and, 21
  tight control of. See Intensified diabetes management
  uncontrolled, 60

Blood vessel damage, 26, 112
Bracelets, diabetes identification, 48
Brain damage, hypoglycemia and, 39
Breakfast. *See* Meal(s)

C

Calories, 82, 84–88, 91, 93, 98, 108
Candy bars, 42, 90
Capsaicin cream, 23
Carbohydrates, 51, 63, 95–96
Certified Diabetes Educators, 101–103
Charts, insulin injection timing, 54
Chemstrip, 14
Children, injections and, 109, 120
Cholesterol, 116
Cloudiness, of regular insulin, 65
Complications, 4–5, 9, 17, 19, 26, 103, 106, 112, 116. *See also* Kidney disease, Nerve disease, Vision problems
Costs of diabetes, 4
Cow's milk, 7
Cortisol, 49

D

Daily routines, for oral medication, 69
Day care, 115
Dentists, 107
Desserts, nonfat, 51
Diabetes Control and Complications Trial (DCCT), 10, 17, 106, 112
Diabetes Forecast, 66, 101
Diascan, 14
Digestion, slowed, 21
Dinner, See Meal(s)
Doses, insulin, 60
  evening, 45
  hyperglycemia and, 31

sickness and, 76
trips and, 16
vomiting and, 75
Drawbacks to blood glucose control, 8

E

Eating, low blood sugar reactions and, 37
Education tips, 99–110
  inforrnation sources, 101
Elderly people, 19, 46, 117, 119
Energy, lack of, 25
Exercise, 12, 56, 60, 82, 84 85, 92–98. *See also* Physical activity
  hypoglycemia and, 41, 45, 95, 97
  records of, 6
  regular, 93
  sexual activity, 98
  walking, 82, 93
Expenses, 15
Eye disease, 9–10, 25–26, 106, 110

F

Fainting, hypoglycemia and, 48
Fasting blood sugar levels, 72, 116
Fat/Fats, 42, 84, 88, 90, 108, 116
Feet, 23, 26
Fevers, 76
Flu. *See* Sickness
Fluids, 31, 77
Flu vaccinations, 81
Forgetting to take, oral medications, 70
Fruit, 87

G

Genetics, 7
Gestational diabetes, 116
Glimepiride, 118
Glipizide GITS, 70

inhaled, 120
injection points, 41, 55–56
injection timing, 54
intentional omission of, 67
lente, 59
NPH, 29–30, 47, 58–59, 78, 87
occupational constraints on use, 66
regimens, 61
regular, 16, 30–31, 34, 40, 56–59,
  61–63, 65, 75–76, 78, 94–96
resistance to, 2, 18, 113
storage of, 64
tips, 53–67
ultralente, 30, 32, 59, 61–62, 87
Insulin-dependent diabetes mellitus,
  2, 5, 20, 71, 106
Insulin injectors, pen-like, 66, 110
Insulin pumps, 15, 61
Insurance, 15
Intensified diabetes management, 19,
  43, 46, 103, 106, 108, 119
Intermediate-acting insulin, 16, 29,
  41, 60, 75, 120

J
Job shift changes, 61
Juice, 34, 42

K
Kidney disease, 9, 13, 18, 26, 106,
  112, 117

L
Lactose, 42
Lancets, 114
Legs insulin injections in, 55
  pain in, 23
Lente insulin, 59
Liquids, 89
Lispro insulin, 16, 30–31, 34, 40,
  56–59, 61–63, 65, 75–76, 78,
  94–96
Long-acting insulin, 16, 29, 41, 60,

75, 79
Lunch, *See* Meal(s)

M
Meal(s), 3, 5, 27, 44, 60
  alcoholic beverages with, 83
  breakfast, 3, 27, 57, 89, 96
  delaying, 31
  dinner, 27, 29, 63
  glycosylated hemoglobin and, 27
  hyperglycemia and, 33
  insulin injection timing and, 54,
    120
  insulin pumps and, 15
  lunch, 27, 57, 62, 66, 78
  plans, 24
  Prandin and, 117
  pre-exercise, 97
  restaurant, 51, 88
  schedule of, 16, 91
Medical help, 77.
Medications, 24
Menstrual periods,
  hyperglycemia and, 36
Meters, blood glucose, 14, 40, 52,
  104
Metformin, 117–118
Microalbuminuria, 13
Milk, 34, 42, 51, 87
Money, saving, 4
Monitoring blood sugar, 114
Morning, blood sugar checks, 35
  hyperglycemia, 30
  hypoglycemia, 41

N
Needlephobia, 109
Nerve disease, 9, 21, 26, 106, 112
Nighttime
  hypoglycemia, 45, 47, 58, 97
  insulin, with oral medication, 72

More Books from the American Diabetes Association

New!
101 Medication Tips for People with Diabetes
Mary Anne Koda-Kimble, PharmD, CDE
Betsy A. Carlisle, PharmD
Lisa Kroon, PharmD

1. What is the difference between regular and lispro insulin?
2. What are the main side effects of the drugs used to treat type 2 diabetes?
3. Will my diabetes medications interact with other drugs I'm taking?
4. My doctor prescribed an "ACE inhibitor." What is this drug? What will it do?

Treating diabetes can get complicated, especially when you consider the bewildering number of medications that must be carefully integrated with diet and exercise. Here you'll find answers to 101 of the most commonly asked questions about diabetes and medication. An indispensable reference for anyone with type 1, type 2, or gestational diabetes.

One Low Price: $14.95
Order #4833-01

New!
101 Nutrition Tips for People with Diabetes
Patti B. Geil, MS, RD, FADA, CDE
Lea Ann Holzmeister, RD, CDE

1. Which type of fiber helps my blood sugar?
2. What do I do if my toddler refuses to eat her meal?
3. If a food is sugar-free, can I eat all I want?

In this latest addition to the best-selling 101 Tips series, co-authors Patti Geil and Lea Ann Holzmeister—experts on nutrition and diabetes—use their professional experience with hundreds of patients over the years to answer the most commonly asked questions about diabetes and nutrition. You'll discover handy tips on meal planning, general nutrition, managing medication and meals, shopping and cooking, weight loss, and more.

One Low Price: $14.95
Order #4828-01

Newly Revised!
101 Tips for Staying Healthy with Diabetes (& Avoiding Complications),
2nd Edition
David S. Schade, MD
and The University of New Mexico Diabetes Care Team

1. Is testing your urine for glucose and ketones an accurate way to measure blood sugar?
2. What's the best way to reduce the pain of frequent finger sticks?
3. Will an insulin pump help you prevent complications?

These are just a few of the more than 110 tips you'll discover in this newly revised second edition of an ADA bestseller. Dozens of other tips—many of them just added—will help you reduce the risk of complications and ensure a healthy life.

One Low Price: $14.95
Order #4810-01

New!
The Diabetes Problem Solver
Nancy Touchette, PhD

Quick: You think you may have diabetic ketoacidosis, a life-threatening condition. What are the symptoms? What should you do first? What are the treatments? How could it have been prevented? *The Diabetes Problem Solver* is the first reference guide that helps you identify and prevent the most common diabetes-related problems you encounter from day-to-day. From hypoglycemia, nerve pain, and foot ulcers to eye disease, depression, and eating disorders, virtually every possible problem is covered. And the solutions are at your fingertips. *The Problem Solver* addresses each problem by answering five crucial questions:
1. What's the problem?
2. Do I have the symptoms?
3. What should I do?
4. What's the best treatment?
You'll find extensive, easy-to-read coverage of just about every diabetes problem you can imagine, and comprehensive flowcharts at the front of the book lead you from symptoms to possible solutions quickly.

One Low Price: $19.95
Order #4825-01

New!
Diabetes Meal Planning on $7 a Day—or Less
Patti B. Geil, MS, RD, FADA, CDE
Tami A. Ross, RD, CDE

You can save money—lots of it—without sacrificing what's most important to you: a healthy variety of great-tasting meals. Learn how to save money by planning meals more carefully, use shopping tips to save money at the grocery store, eat at your favorite restaurants economically, and much more. Each of the 100 quick and easy recipes includes cost-per-serving and complete nutrition information to help you create a more cost-conscious, healthy meal plan.

One Low Price: $12.95
Order #4711-01

New!
Meditations on Diabetes
Catherine Feste

Modern medicine has come full circle to realize again what ancient healers knew: that illness affects both the body and the soul. Cathy Feste has lived with diabetes for 40 years, so she knows the physical, emotional, and spiritual challenges that come with diabetes. With every turn of the page you'll discover reassuring advice and insight in daily meditations from the author's journals with a little help from her friends, such as Ralph Waldo Emerson, Eleanor Roosevelt, Helen Keller, and many others.

One Low Price: $13.95
Order #4820-01

When Diabetes Hits Home
Wendy Satin Rapaport, LCSW, PsyD

A reassuring exploration of the full spectrum of emotional issues you and your family may struggle with throughout your lives. You'll learn how to cope with the initial period of anger and anxiety at diagnosis, develop your spiritual self and discover the meaning of living with a chronic disease, address the changes all families go through and learn how to cope with them emotionally, and much more.

One Low Price: $19.95
Order #4818-01

The Uncomplicated Guide to Diabetes Complications
Edited by Marvin E. Levin, MD
and Michael A. Pfeifer, MD

Thorough, comprehensive chapters cover everything you need to know about preventing and treating diabetes complications—in simple language that anyone can understand. All major complications and special concerns are covered, including kidney disease, heart disease, obesity, eye disease and blindness, impotence and sexual disorders, hypertension and stroke, neuropathy and vascular disease, and more.

One Low Price: $18.95
Order #4814-01

Women & Diabetes
Laurinda M. Poirier, RN, MPH, CDE
Katherine M. Coburn, MPH

A woman's life is complex enough with all the roles that she plays during her lifetime. Diabetes compounds the complexity and challenges a woman mentally, physically, and spiritually. This book, written by two health professionals—one of whom has diabetes—offers special thoughts to help you move through life with confidence.

Nonmember: $14.95
Member: $13.95
Order #4907-01

Caring for the Diabetic Soul
Simple solutions for coping with the psychological challenges of diabetes.

Nonmember: $9.95
Member: $8.95
Order #4815-01

Winning with Diabetes
Inspiring true stories of people who live life to the fullest, despite having diabetes.

One Low Price: $12.95
Order #4824-01

Dear Diabetes Advisor
Michael A. Pfeifer, MD, CDE

Solid, no-nonsense answers to commonsense questions about diabetes.

Nonmember: $9.95
Member: $8.95
Order #4813-01

Best-seller!
American Diabetes Association Complete Guide to Diabetes
A thorough guide packed with ideas, tips, and techniques for dealing with
all types of diabetes.

Nonmember: $19.95
Member: $15.95
Order #4809-01

Revised Best-seller!
Type 2 Diabetes: Your Healthy Living Guide, 2nd Edition
A thorough guide to staying healthy with type 2 diabetes.

Nonmember: $16.95
Member: $14.95
Order #4804-01

New!
The Great Chicken Cookbook for People with Diabetes
Beryl M. Marton

Now you can have chicken any way you want it—and healthy too! More
than 150 great-tasting, low-fat chicken recipes in all, including baked
chicken, braised chicken, chicken casseroles, grilled chicken, rolled and
stuffed chicken, chicken soups, chicken stir-fry, chicken with pasta, and
many more.

One Low Price: $16.95
Order #4627-01

New!
The New Soul Food Cookbook for People with Diabetes
Fabiola Demps Gaines, RD, LD
Roneice Weaver, RD, LD

Dig into sensational low-fat recipes from the first African-American cookbook for people with diabetes. More than 150 recipes in all, including shrimp jambalaya, fried okra, orange sweet potatoes, corn muffins, apple crisp, and many more.

One Low Price: $14.95
Order #4623-01

New!
The Diabetes Snack Munch Nibble Nosh Book
Ruth Glick

Choose from 150 low-sodium, low-fat snacks and mini-meals, such as pizza puffs, mustard pretzels, apple-cranberry turnovers, bread puzzle, cinnamon biscuits and pecan buns, alphabet letters, banana pops, and many others. Special features include recipes for one or two and snack ideas for hard-to-please kids. Nutrient analyses, preparation times, and exchanges are included with every recipe.

One Low Price: $14.95
Order Code: #4622-01

The ADA Guide to Healthy Restaurant Eating
Hope S. Warshaw, MMSc, RD, CDE

Finally! One book with all the facts you need to eat out intelligently—whether you're enjoying burgers, pizza, bagels, pasta, or burritos at your favorite restaurant. Special features include more than 2,500 menu items from more than 50 major restaurant chains, complete nutrition information for every menu item, restaurant pitfalls and strategies for defensive restaurant dining, and much more.

One Low Price: $13.95
Order #4819-01

About the American Diabetes Association

The American Diabetes Association is the nation's leading voluntary health organization supporting diabetes research, information, and advocacy. Founded in 1940, the Association provides services to communities across the country. Its mission is to prevent and cure diabetes and to improve the lives of all people affected by diabetes.

For more than 50 years, the American Diabetes Association has been the leading publisher of comprehensive diabetes information for people with diabetes and the health care professionals who treat them. Its huge library of practical and authoritative books for people with diabetes covers every aspect of self care—cooking and nutrition, fitness, weight control, medications, complications, emotional issues, and general self care. The Association also publishes books and medical treatment guides for physicians and other health care professionals.

Membership in the Association is available to health care professionals and people with diabetes and includes subscriptions to one or more of the Association's periodicals. People with diabetes receive *Diabetes Forecast*, the nation's leading health and wellness magazine for people with diabetes. Health care professionals receive one or more of the Association's five scientific and medical journals.

For more information, please call toll-free:

Questions about diabetes: 1-800-DIABETES
Membership, people with diabetes: 1-800-806-7801
Membership, health professionals: 1-800-232-3472
Free catalog of ADA books: 1-800-232-6733
Visit us on the Web: www.diabetes.org
Visit us at our Web bookstore: merchant.diabetes.org